Chinese Horology

MADE EASY

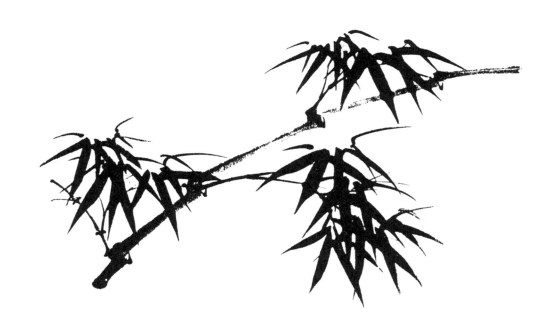

BY

MAOSHING NI, C.A.

PHOTO BY KATHRYN LANIER, C.A.

DISCLAIMER

The contents of this book are intended to be a study guide for learning. This book is not intended to replace consultation with your doctor or to be used in self-treatment.

The author and publisher of this book shall not be held liable for any harm which may occur by misapplication of the information in this book.

Published by:
SevenStar Communications
13315 Washington Boulevard, Suite 200
Los Angeles, California 90066 USA

The paper used in this publication meets the minimum requirements of the American National Standard for Information Sciences Permanence of Paper for Printed Library Materials, ANSI 239.48- 1984.

First Printing: November, 1986
Second Printing: September, 1991
Third Printing: June, 1994
Fourth Printing: October, 1995
Fifth Printing: February, 2001

Library of Congress Cataloging-in-Publication Data

Ni, Maoshing.
   Chinese herbology made easy / by Maoshing Ni ; photo by Kathryn Lanier.
      201, [13] p., [1] leaf of plates : ill. ; 28 cm.
   Includes indexes.
   Bibliography: p.[203].
   ISBN 0-937064- 12-2
   1. Herbs- -Therapeutic use. 2. Materia Medica- -China. 3. Medicinal plants- -China.
I. Title.
RM222.H33 1986   89-63041
615 / .321 19   CIP

DEDICATION

Dedicated to the ancient masters that made this knowledge available and to those that courageously embark onto this path to better themselves and the world.

ACKNOWLEDGEMENTS

I wish to thank my father, Master Ni, Hua-Ching for his guidance, support and opportunity and to My teacher Dr. Jiang Jian Fu for her unselfishness in sharing with me her deep understanding of Chinese Medicine. I am indebted to my mother Lily for her untiring nurturing, my brother Daoshing for his encouragement and my sister in law Sum Yee for her help. A special thanks goes to my dearest friend, Kathryn Lanier, who I could always count on when it became difficult. I am grateful for her endless help and support that made this book a reality. And to all my teachers and friends who helped me, and continue to do so, along my path of growth, I sincerely thank them all from my heart.

ABOUT THE AUTHOR

Maoshing Ni, born into a family of medical traditions as the thirty-eighth generation of traditional Chinese healers, began his training early in life. He studied intensively with his father and many other teachers in the subject of Chinese Medicine, martial arts, Tai Chi Chuan, Taoism and other related arts in China. He attended schools in China and the United States and received his advanced degrees and license as an acupuncturist. He has worked in various hospitals and clinics here and in China. Presently, he is in private practice in Los Angeles and lectures extensively at acupuncture colleges on various subjects of Chinese Medicine and dietary therapy. He also teaches Tai Chi Chuan and other energy exercises. His goal is to make Chinese Medicine widely available in the West, and someday, to see it not only as Chinese Medicine, but as universal medicine!

PREFACE

When I was six years old, I lived in Taiwan, a small island the size of Vermont, off the coast of mainland China where 12 million people lived. Like many small, densely populated areas, the only way to expand was upward. As our house began adding fourth and fifth stories that summer, I was kept out of the house amidst of the construction. At the time my father was a busy doctor practicing Chinese Medicine and my mother was an elementary school teacher teaching summer school. Thus, it was the first and only summer that I had a complete reign over my activities, and of course, I took full advantage of it.

One July morning after my mother left for school, my brother and I decided to be adventurous and go up to the roof top where the construction site was. After curiously rummaging through the building materials we chased each other around with sticks that we pretended were broad swords. As we fought and chased each other toward the edge of the building, my brother, whom I was chasing after, made a swift turn near the edge and I just headed straight over the edge and plunged over 40 feet onto the asphalt-surfaced street down below.

There I laid unconscious in a puddle of blood, and will to live must have somehow managed to keep my spirit from abandoning me. After about 20 minutes I was finally "discovered" by a soap salesman who was advertising with his P.A. system from his truck. He carried me in his truck and drove around the block 3 times announcing me through his P.A. system. All this time, I had remained unconscious and covered with blood. My father finally came out, and I woke up the instant that he picked me up. He then took me inside the house and put me on his treatment table as the blood continued to gush from all over my body. I was ghostly pale and my blood pressure dropped rapidly from the massive bleeding. I was told later that everyone just sighed and thought I was going to die. A neighbor suggested that I should be rushed to the hospital which was 40 miles away, but my father just shook his head and refused. He quickly examined me and then sprinkled some herbal powder on my chin and all over my body and forced me to swallow some herbs. Magically, a few minutes later he returned to find the bleeding completely stopped and my blood pressure normalized. He evacuated the room and left me alone as I slowly drifted into sleep. Next day I was able to get up and resume most of my usual activities, but for the next two weeks I practically lived on herbs. So terrified was my mother that she insisted on taking me to the hospital despite disagreement from my father. At the hospital I went through every possible exam, x-rays and blood test there was and everything turned up negative. As for my bones, they found not a single fracture anywhere in my body, even on my chin where I had actually landed.

Of course my father restrained my activities after that and my following summers would never be the same again.

Today, a tiny scar under my chin serves to remind me of the incident and how I owe my life to Chinese Medicine.

I have since taken up the study and practice of Chinese Medicine, especially herbology, which is as complex and yet essential as any treatment modality in Chinese Medicine.

When learning Chinese herbology, do not be frustrated if the subject seems overwhelming. Try to integrate it into yourself and your life. No book can be the absolute authority on the subject, only you, the practitioner who have learned it through the sufferings of yourself and your patients, will truly know and understand its nature. An old

Chinese doctor once told me how, when he was younger, he had studied many books on Chinese Medicine for 3 years and was confident that there was no disease he could not cure. He then practiced for three years and realized that no book was useful and complete. This is not to say that a student doesn't have to study books, but rather, all books merely provide a foundation, a basis for one to integrate further knowledge and experience. This is especially true in medicine where every situation can be so different and thus require adaptive abilities and knowledge.

Learning about herbs is like learning about ourselves. Every herb is uniquely different in function, just like each of us has limitless possibilities. How to bring out the actions of each herb is a matter of knowing how to realize our many potentials to the fullest.

Maoshing Ni
September, 1986

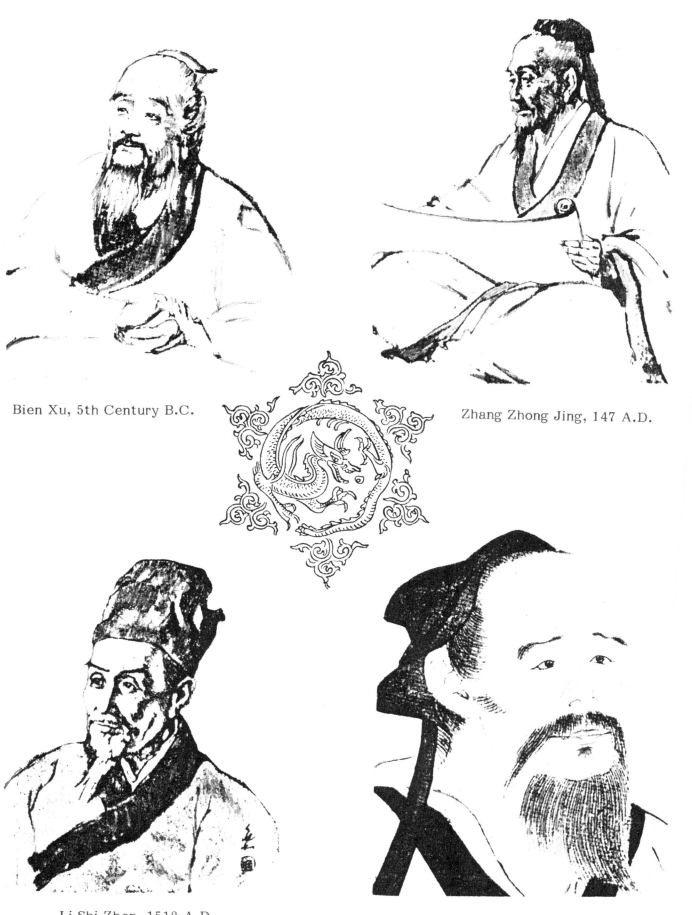

Bien Xu, 5th Century B.C.

Zhang Zhong Jing, 147 A.D.

Li Shi Zhen, 1518 A.D.

Hua Tuo, 141 A.D.

CONTENTS

LIST OF TABLES

DEVELOPMENT OF CHINESE HERBOLOGY

The Origin

On the great Yellow River Plateau of China, Shen Nong, the tribal chief, said to have existed around 2700 B.C., was doing his routine gathering and studying of herbal substance one day when he encountered 70 poisonous substances. He experimented by ingesting these substances to determine their therapeutic values. Through diligent and laborious efforts like this, Shen Nong recorded in writing the very first book on Traditional Chinese herbal medicine - *The Classic of Materia Medica (Shen Nong Ben Cao Jing)*, which describes about 365 healing substances. These include 252 from plant source, 46 from minerals and 67 from animal source. In actuality, the work was compiled around 206 B.C. and is a direct reflection of all the knowledge and practical experiences accumulated on the subject before the Han era (2nd century B.C.). This book laid down the foundation for the development of Chinese Herbal medicine in the next two millennia that followed.

Then came the Yellow Emperor (2697 - 2597 B.C.), a wise and virtuous man who defeated the invasion of a barbaric tribe to unite all the tribes in China into one nation for the first time. He was a very kind and compassionate leader whose concern for the welfare of his citizens outweighed his own. Ever searching for knowledge to properly guide his people, a famous dialogue took place between the Yellow Emperor and his physician, Qi Bo, a famous healer and scholar of that era. The recorded conversation between the Yellow Emperor and Qi Bo revealed such subjects as human anatomy and physiology, etiology of disease, pathology, diagnosis and treatment, disease prevention, health preservation, man and nature, application of Taoist theories of Yin and Yang, Five elements, acupuncture and more. These conversations were the contents of a monumental work called the *Yellow Emperor's Classics of Internal Medicine (Huang Di Nei Jing)* written during the Warring States era around 305 -204 B.C.. This Classic text which is still in use today is no doubt the world's earliest and most comprehensive book on medicine. In it, the emphasis is placed on disease prevention, as illustrated by the following quote:

> *The sages of ancient times emphasized not the treatment of diseases, rather the prevention of its occurrence. To administer medicine to disease which has already developed and to suppress revolts which have already begun is comparable to the behavior of one who begins to dig a well after he has become thirsty or one who begins to forge weapons after he engaged in battle. Would these actions not be too late?*

> *- Su Wen, Yellow Emperor's Classics*

First Millennia

Around the third century A.D., a famous physician named Zhang Zhong Jing witnessed the tragedy of an infectious disease which took the lives of two thirds of his clan. Out of grief for his clan and frustration over the limitations of medicine against such diseases, he became determined to conquer these shortcoming of medicine at that time. Years of dedicated study, observation, and experience lead to his writing of the *Shang Han lun (A Discussion of Cold Induced Disease)* and *Jin Gui Yao Lun (Synopsis of*

1

Prescriptions of the Golden Chamber). These classical books became the basis for prescription/formula writing in Chinese Medicine. Even today his books remain essential in diagnosis and treatment of infectious diseases.

Taoism, the Foundation

Taoism is a philosophy of universal governing laws and an integral way of life. It is the cornerstone of Chinese Medicine. The theory of Yin and Yang is the rudimentary principle of all Chinese thinking and Medicine. A quote from the *Yellow Emperor's Classics* properly illustrates this:

> *Yin/Yang is the Way of heaven and earth,*
> *The fundamental principle of the myriad things,*
> *The father and mother of change and transformation,*
> *The root of inception and destruction.*
>   *- Su Wen, Yellow Emperor's Classics*

Chinese Medicine was only one of many cultivated arts acquired by the ancient Taoists. Besides mastering Chinese Medicine, their studies also included subjects such as Astrology, Geomancy, physiognomy, palmistry, I-Ching, Internal Alchemy, Martial Arts, Tai Chi Chuan, Life Charting, etc. Especially the art of Internal Alchemy which will lead to our next physician, Tao Hong Jing.

Tao Hong Jing was a well known Taoist and herbalist living around 452 A.D. He was extremely interested in the science of alchemy – a practice involving making elixirs for immortality by chemical synthesis, a process that predated modern chemistry by two millennia. His contribution to Chinese Medicine was the restructuring and editing of the original *Classics of Materia Medica (Shen Nong Ben Cao Jing)* into categories of substances by Kingdoms, such as plant kingdom, mineral kingdom, animal kingdom, insect/fish kingdom, vegetable/fruit kingdom. He also added to the whole body of herb entries for a total of 730 substances. This system of organization prevailed a thousand years afterwards where Li Shi Zhen also used it in his work of the *Grand Materia Medica (Ben Cao Gung Mu)*, in 1590 A.D.

Government Support

By the Tang Dynasty (618 A.D.), the government took the task of compiling the first official Pharmacopeia in history. In this book, titled *Newly Revised Materia Medica (Xin Xiu Ben Cao)*, there are about 844 illustrated entries. It is considered to be the earliest officially published pharmacopoeia in the world.

The Sung Dynasty (960 – 1279 A.D.) brought further expansion to the Materia Medica. With many inventions and the advancement in printing, it greatly facilitated the dissemination of information to the masses. One person responsible for the expansion of Herbal medicine at this time was Tang Shen Wei. A man with the reputation of bringing the dead back to life. He spent years gathering and compiling information on Herbal medicine and eventually wrote a book called *Classified Materia Medica (Zheng Lei Ben Cao)*. This book was valuable in that it listed 1,746 substances with directions and preparations for use. It laid a solid foundation for the development of the knowledge of the Materia medica (Ben Cao) for the next 500 years.

Second Millennia

As time went on, more and more knowledge was accumulated and added to the body of the Materia Medica. The most massive undertaking of them all was the book, *Grand Materia Medica (Ben Cao Gang Mu, 1590 A.D.)* sometimes referred to as the *Compendium of Materia Medica*. Compiled by Li Shi Zhen, this book in 52 volumes was the most comprehensive Materia Medica book in the world. It took the author 30 years of persistent researching, gathering, identifying and consolidating, and resulted in 1,892 substances with more than 1000 illustrations, over 10,000 prescriptions. Each substance also had a detailed description of its appearance, properties, method of collection, preparation and use. This monumental book was later translated into 14 different languages and is still in print in those languages today. Li Shi Zhen could not afford or find anyone to publish his gigantic work while he was alive and died a disheartened man.

The Modern Era

The 20th century saw a revival of the more natural traditional medicine. This arose out of increasing discontentment towards the more conventional medicine. The knowledge of herbal medicine has become prevalent and its use has accelerated to an all-time-high in popularity. In China, many scientific studies have been conducted on the biochemical/pharmaceutical functions of herbs to satisfy the curiosity of its scientific counterpart in the west and to aid the advancement of medical treatment. Hence, the expansion of the Materia Medica to a total of 5,767 entries by the Jiangsu College of New Medicine in China in 1977, is not at all surprising.

INTRODUCTION

THE WHOLISTIC APPROACH

In the midst of increasing dissatisfaction with the conventional orthodox medicine, many people in the Western world are desperately seeking alternative solutions to their health problems. The most promising of that alternative solution is Chinese Medicine, which is the oldest medical tradition in human civilization. For the one billion people on the other side of this planet, Chinese Medicine is THE medicine and not the alternative. The fact that it is thousands of years old and still widely used up to date is testament to its effectiveness, having withstood the test of time.

The ancient Chinese perceived everything as whole. They saw the universe that they lived in as one, and they were part of that oneness. They did not try to separate things, but rather, they kept everything in their natural wholesome state. They observed the changes that took place around them. The changes in the positions of the stars, the changes in the seasons and the weather and the changes in the face of the earth. With observations and sensitivity they were able to correlate the human body with the universe. The volcanic eruptions of the earth, rumbling earthquakes, thunderstorms and lightening, tornadoes, drought, heat waves, rain and sun can all be reflected in the human body.

These similar changes occur in the human body as seasons of birth, growth, development, maturity and cessation; as in extreme temperature reactions in high fever, chills, sweating; as eruptions to expel as in vomiting and diarrhea, and as sudden as a tornado in convulsions and strokes. Through these correlations, a principle was perceived that the human organism is not all that much different from its surroundings, the macrocosm. The laws that governed his surroundings also applied to him. So he formulated patterns of these changes, and even as everything changes, the law of these changes remains unchangeable.

Unlike the modern medicine which is becoming increasing mechanical, Chinese Medicine still maintains its unique qualities of individuality, adaptability and effectiveness.

A practitioner of Chinese Medicine sees a patient as a whole, and he realizes that every individual is different, and thus he will respond differently to a condition that may be labelled as the same in conventional medicine. He realizes that a condition may change from one day to the next, from one hour to the next, and even from one minute to the next minute. Because he is flexible and adaptive to efficiently provide the body's needs, he is then able to deal with each condition individually and effectively. This is why Chinese medicine is able to thrive into the nuclear era of 20th century.

While modern medicine is just starting to recognize the mental and physical connection of diseases, thousands of years ago, these ancient healers knew that the body was more than just physical. They knew that the body consisted of the mental, physical and spiritual aspects that exert influence on one another. Hence, a modality was developed to integrate all three aspects of the human body.

Herbology is the core of treatment in Chinese Medicine. By utilizing substances together in their whole form in accurate formulations, effectiveness will be maximized and side effects minimized. This is contrary to

4

conventional medicine that extracts or synthesizes certain active chemicals which often time produce drastic side effects due to their partiality.

YIN - YANG

The ancient Taoist sages described the universe and their surroundings through a concept that is still very valid today. That concept is Yin and Yang, which is the rudimentary principle in Chinese Medicine. The concept provides a basis for the analysis of all phenomena and things into complementary groups, whether it's applied to nature or the human body.

It was stated in the Yellow Emporer's Classics that "the universe is an expression of the interplay and alternation of the two activities of Yin and Yang." There is no aspects of life to which the activities of Yin and Yang do not apply. Yin and Yang have no absolute definitions, rather, they are defined in terms relative to each other. In nature, there are no thing or phenomena that is absolutely Yin or Yang. Take an example of the basic unit of the universe, the atom. As miniscule as the atom, it is composed of two opposite yet complementary parts, the proton which is positively charged, and the electron which is negatively charged. Yin and Yang represent two broad categories of complements that include the polar aspects of every phenomena such as negativity and positivity, constructive and destructive, beginning and ending, active and passive, etc. These correspondences can continue ad infinitum.

When applied to the human organism, the material aspect, the flesh, the blood, and the bones are considered to be Yin; and the functional aspect, the metabolism, the circulation and the Qi are considered to be Yang. In disease state, it becomes even more obvious. In Chinese Medicine, disease is the result of an imbalance of Yin and Yang in the body. Conditions manifesting Heat and Cold signs and symptoms are considered Yang and Yin conditions respectively. However, Cold condition in one instance may transform into Heat condition in the next instance, and vice versa, depending on the situation and causative factors involved. Disease is ever changing, what affects one person may manifest differently in another. The principle of Yin - Yang is a direct reflection of these changes. In medicine, this principle enables the practioner to grasp the dynamics of disease course, hence, he becomes more capable in his diagnosis and treatment of diseases.

The essence of Chinese Medicine is to help one seek balance of Yin and Yang within himself and harmony with his environment.

THE FIVE PHASES (OR ELEMENTS)

The theory of the Five Phases was formulated by the ancients to describe the cyclical phases of energy evolution in the universe. The Five Phases, sometimes translated as the "Five Elements", is both dynamic and static. The static aspect applies to the basic material spheres of the universe. These elements, both literal and symbolic, are represented by wood, fire, earth, metal and water elements. These elements, or energies, follow the Law of Changes, transforms into one another in a cyclical, orderly manner. The balance is sustained through Cycles of Creation and Destruction of the elements.

It is not hard to visualize the Creation Cycle of the elements. The wood element which represents the beginning, the birth of energies, derives its origin from the "mother of all living things", the water element. The water, which is Yin (inactive) in nature, gives support to the Yang (active) which is functional and characteristic of life. Thus, the Creation Cycle draws from the water element, but begins with the wood element. Rubbing two pieces of wood together creates fire, the fire burns the wood into ashes, which becomes the earth. The earth produces metal ores which is then melted down into liquid, the water, and the water germinates wood. The cycle is repeated over again without cease.

In the Destructive Cycle, the same water element that gives birth to life can also inhibit growth. The water puts out fire. The fire melts down the metal. The metal is forged into an axe which is used to cut apart the wood. The wood infiltrates the earth with its roots and the earth contains the water with valleys or dams. The term "destructive cycle" does not literally mean destroying the elements, rather, it denotes control of one element on another to maintain the energy balance.

In physiology and pathology, we can see the energy and disease evolution occuring within the body through this cyclical phase. Each organ corresponds to one element. A balance is established where each organ supports another organ and controls a third organ. Furthermore, it also receives nourishment from its source organ. Therefore, it is easy to see that a disease state involving one organ may affect other associate organs through this pattern of energy transformation.

The correspondence of the Five Phases to the internal organs are as follows: The wood corresponds to the Liver and the Gall bladder, the fire to the Heart, Small intestines, Pericardium and the Sanjiao, the earth to the Spleen and the Stomach, the metal to the Lungs and the Large intestines, and the water to the Kidneys and the Bladder.

THE FOUR ENERGIES

In Chinese Medicine, each herb is said to have a particular energy of its own. It has either Hot, Cold, Warm or Cool energy. There is also an intermediary energy called neutral in which is neither Hot nor Cold. These energies draw their definition from the body's response after taking the herbs. In general, Chinese Medicine divides disease into two types, Cold and Heat, or in essence, Yin and Yang.

The Heat type manifests symptoms such redness, swelling, fever, thirst, scanty concentrated urine. The causes of the Heat type are numerous. Examples include what are called a Warm or Hot type of pathogens invading the body, or that the body Yang is in excess. Another reason for manifesting Heat symptoms is arising from deficiency of the body's Yin which causes imbalance resulting in relative excess of body's Yang. For victims suffering from Heat type of conditions, the treatment principle will simply be to Cool or introduce Cold herbs to counteract the Heat. Because of different causes of the Heat types of conditions, the treatment principle varies accordingly. If the pathogen invades from the outside of the body, it should then be expelled from the body. For one that has excess of Yang energy, one needs to be subdued, whereas relative Heat condition arising from insufficiency of Yin should be nourished with Yin tonics.

Chills in the extremities, and the body, copious, clear urine, pale face, and so on are all part of the symptomatology of the Cold type of condition. The Cold type is exactly opposite to the Hot type. The cause again varies such as pathogenic Cold entering the body from the Exterior, or a relative Yin Excess in the body, or because of an insufficiency of Yang in the body. The treatment principles, thus, are very similar to that of the Heat type in that it differs according to the cause, whether to dispel, to subdue or to tonify. Therefore, with the Cold type of condition, one must utilize Warm or Hot herbs to counteract the Cold.

THE FIVE TASTES

The physical sensation of taste has its significance in Chinese Medicine. In Chinese Medicine, it is classified into five taste, although in the text you will actually find seven tastes. These five taste are sour, sweet, bitter, pungent and salty. The other two are bland, which falls under the sweet category, and astringent, which goes under the sour category.

When a substance such as a food or an herb goes into the gastrointestinal tract to be digested, the sour taste is said to be absorbed by the Liver and Gall Bladder, the bitter taste by the Heart and Small Intestines, the sweet taste by the Spleen and Stomach, the pungent taste by the Lungs and Large Intestines, and the salty taste by the Kidney and Bladder. Therefore, foods and herbs with different energies and tastes are assimilated into the body to nourish different organs. Take the example of someone with digestive difficulties as in a weakness of Spleen and Stomach; he or she often likes to eat sweets. Contrary to Western medicine, in that those with digestive weakness are advised against sweets intake, Chinese Medicine utilizes herbs that are actually slightly sweet to strengthen the weakness of Spleen and Stomach.

Pungent is a taste that has functions of dispersing, invigorating, and promoting circulation. Its function of dispersing is mainly used to disperse pathogens from the Exterior of the body. It is seen, for example, in common cold and flu. Its function of invigorating is to promote circulation of Qi, blood and body fluid. In Chinese Medicine, disease is the result of stagnation, therefore, herbs that have this pungent taste will promote and invigorate circulation of the Qi, blood and body fluids. Pathological condition of stagnation can be seen as local pain, irregular menstruation, painful menstruation, edema, tumors, and so on. The pungent taste, because of its dispersing quality also acts to open the pores and promote sweating. This is a way to expel the pathogen from the body. An example of a pungent tasting herb is ginger (Rizoma Zingiberis).

Sour taste has absorbing, consolidating, and astringent functions. It functions in stopping abnormal discharge of body fluids and substances as in condition of excessive perspiration, diarrhea, seminal emission, spermatorrhea, enuresis and so on. An example of a sour herb is Chinese sour plum (Fructus Mume).

Astringent taste falls under the sour taste category and its actions are very similar to that of the sour taste.

Bitter tasting herbs have the action of drying dampness and dispersing. So bitter aids conditions like dampness and edema. Its function of dispersing obstruction can be utilized in cough due to Qi stagnation and so forth. Examples of bitter tasting herbs are rhubarb (Rizoma Rhei) and apricot kernel (Semen Armeniacae).

7

Salty taste has the function of softening and dissolving hardenings. It also moistens and lubricates the intestines. Body symptoms such as lumps, nodes, masses, cysts and so on can be softened and dissolved by salty substances. Example can be seen in goiter which is treated by seaweed, a representative of salty herbs. Also, in cases of constipation, one can drink salt water to lubricate and promote evacuation.

Sweet taste has the action of tonifying, harmonizing and decelerating. In cases of fatigue or deficiency, sweet substances have a reinforcing and strengthening action. Deficiencies may be resulted in different aspects of the body, such as insufficiency of Qi, blood, Yin or Yang. Various organs may suffer from weakness also. This is why one is drawn to sweet when he or she is experiencing low energy. Sweet taste is also used to decelerate, which means to relax. It is used in conditions of acute pain to help relax and hence, ease the pain. Sweet substances and herbs can harmonize as an antidote or counter balance undesirable effects from some herbs. Example of sweet tasting herbs are licorice (Radix Glycerriza) and Chinese dates (Fructus Jujube).

Bland taste falls in under the sweet taste category. It tends to be diuretic, promotes urination and relieves edema. An example of a bland tasting herbs is corn silk (Stylus Zeae Mays).

There are obvious ways in which one can relate Chinese Herbology to treatment of a patient. For example, herbs that are yellow in color tend to enter the Spleen and Stomach meridians and act on the digestive system. Therefore, we can see from the theory of Five Elements or Phases that the color yellow corresponds to the element Earth, and the organs of the Earth are Spleen and Stomach. The part of the herb also plays a significant role, such as a seed will tend to descend and lubricate the intestine and a flower will tend to affect the upper part of the body, especially the head. Whereas the herbs that are branches tend to be used for problems of the extremities, herbs from the insect family are used to treat obstruction in the channels and collaterals affecting mobility. The herbs from the mineral family such as shells and stones are used to calm down on an Ascending condition.

ZANG FU (Chinese view of the internal organs)

Chinese view of the internal organs differs drastically from the Western perception. It describes the organs in terms of their "energetic" functions as opposed to their "physical function". In Chinese Medicine, every internal organ is connected to numerous channels and collaterals which supply the energy and nourishment to the organs for functioning. Thus, herbs derive their effectiveness from the channels which they enter, or in effect, the organs that they act on.

The organs are classified into two types: the hollow organs or the solid organs. The hollow organs are more functional and considered Yang; the solid organs are more substantial and considered Yin.

The Yin organs are referred to as the Zang organs. Zang (the solid organs) in Chinese Medicine actually denotes "store", whereas Fu (the hollow organs) denotes "house" or "palace". The Zangs and Fus function within the body in pairs, with one Zang organ as the Yin polarity of one phase in the cycle of energy evolution in the body, and one Fu organ as its complementary

8

Yang polarity. They are interdependent of each other in that the Zang organs need the energy of the Fu organs to properly transform and store essence. Similarly, the Fu's function of transportation is provided by the transformed energy from the Zangs.

Zang Organs

The **Liver**, according to Chinese Medicine, is considered "the general" of the five Zang organs. Thus, it is just like a general in an army in that when the general is strong, the troops are not easily defeated. Therefore, a strong liver will mean a strong constitution. On the other hand, if the liver is weak then one becomes vulnerable to disease. The liver stores blood and maintains a smoothness of Qi flow. The liver, just like a person, does not like restrictions. It likes to be free flowing and carefree. Thus, in situations where there is emotional stress and pressure, the liver will act up and cause a lot of problems. The liver controls tendons and opens to the eyes; thus, when the liver is affected, in Chinese Medicine, one may become very tense and spastic and manifest eye ailments.

The **Heart** is the supreme master of the organs. It governs the blood vessels and promotes the smooth circulation of blood throughout the body. It also houses and the Spirit. The Spirit, in Chinese Medicine, has different levels, including the ability to comprehend, remember, think and respond. It is also responsible for awareness and realization. Thus, when the heart is affected, one will manifest symptoms such as palpitations, chest pains, poor memory, insomnia, and mental disorders.

The **Spleen** is responsible for the assimilation and transportation of nutrients throughout the body. Therefore, a weakness in spleen will often cause indigestion, malnutrition, and a thin body. It governs the muscles, the extremities, and the flesh (either too much as in obesity or not enough as in thinness). Heavy limbs often suggests a spleen disharmony. The spleen also produces blood and is responsible for maintaining the health of the blood vessels. Thus, weak spleen is often manifested as anemic conditions or weakness in blood vessels causing bleeding and bruising.

The **Lungs** govern respiration; thus, they are responsible for taking the energy from the environment to feed the body. Lung problems may include asthma, cough, and various respiratory dysfunctions. The lungs also govern the circulation of the body fluids. Thus, if the lungs become affected we may see edema, emaciation, drying and shriveling of the skin. Lungs also govern the skin and the pores. Therefore, conditions of acute skin lesions have to do with the lungs. The associated sensory organ is the nose.

The **Kidneys** store the essence and regulate fluid metabolism. The essence has three purposes: to promote growth and development, to absorb the essence from food and produce blood, and to reproduce. Thus, a weakness in kidneys will manifest as poor growth and development, anemia, impotence, infertility, edema, and fluid metabolism disorders. The kidneys govern the bones, marrow, hair, and ears. So as the aging process goes, the bones become soft or brittle, hearing ability diminishes, and hair becomes thin or brittle; kidney weakness is indicated.

The **Pericardium**, in Chinese Medicine, is responsible for protecting the heart. However, many conditions of heart disharmony can also include the pericardium, such as anxiety and mental disorders.

Fu organs

The **Gall Bladder** is responsible for making decisions of when certain organs function, and when they rest. Disharmony in the gall bladder may manifest as indecisiveness and inability to rest, as in insomnia.

The **Stomach** governs digestion. Disharmonies manifest as lack of appetite, indigestion, vomiting, nausea, and so forth.

The **Small Intestine** separates the pure and turbid aspects of fluids and transports it to various parts of the body. It receives processed food from the stomach and transport it to the large intestines. Thus, diarrhea, constipation, and urinary disorder are some of the symptoms of small intestine disharmony.

The **Large Intestine** is responsible for transportation of waste product out of the body and governs the rectum. Thus, constipation, dysentery, diarrhea and hemorrhoids, are manifestations of large intestine disharmony.

The **Bladder** stores and excretes water. Disharmonies in the bladder can be seen in edema and urinary disorders.

The **San Jiao** (triple heater) is not an organ, rather, it is the three cavities of the trunk. The classics described the Sanjiao as an organ without form. Its function is in maintaining a communication with all the organs and all the cavities of the body while promoting circulation. It is intimately associated with fluid circulation through the three Jiaos; thus, problems with water metabolism can result from dysfunction of San Jiao. When the triple warmer is affected, almost all organs will be affected.

CAUSES OF DISEASE

There are external, internal, and miscellaneous causes of diseases in Chinese Medicine. The external causes mainly result from changes in environmental factors such as wind, damp, heat, summer heat, and dryness. These can all affect an individual who is either deficient or unable to adapt to the changes of environment. Thus, these environmental pathogens can then harm the body. For example, common cold is usually due to pathogenic wind. Acute inflammations, infections, burns, and eye diseases can be manifestations of heat. Cold manifests as pain or chills. When exposed to the summer sun for long periods of time, such symptoms as fever, sweating, and irritability may result. Dampness may occur as seasonal pains in the back and joints. Extreme dryness in weather may cause problems with lungs such as asthma and bronchitis.

Internal causes are mainly emotional imbalances. Joy, anger, worry, grief, fear, melancholy, and so forth can all affect the body's functions. For example, extreme anger can injure the liver and cause liver problems. Extreme joy can cause heart problems. Constant worrying can injure the spleen. Grief can affect the lungs. Fear and fright can weaken the kidneys.

Other miscellaneous factors that cause disharmony are due to irregular and improper eating habits, overexertion, overwork, traumas, injuries, and so on. In reality, the causes of disease are not necessarily isolated all the time. There is usually more than one cause of the disharmony as a whole.

HOW TO USE THIS BOOK

Chinese herbology is a very complex subject for the student to master. There are bulk information now available on each individual herb, however, one can choose to memorize all the information about each herb and yet not understand or use it correctly. This book will help the student to properly learn the subject of Chinese Herbology. It is presented in the most simple way and yet still retaining the essential information. It is by no means a comprehensive text on the subject, but it does provide the foundation for Chinese Herbology. The students are encouraged to look up books listed in the bibliography section for more information on each herb.

You will find that the herbs in this book are laid out in chart form, so one can glance easily over the chart to obtain the essential information on each herb. It is important to understand how these herbs are categorized and why they are put together in one category and not the other.

Prior to each category there is an introduction to the categories. It is crucial that one studies the introduction thoroughly to gain understanding before proceeding to learn about each individual herb. Within, it defines why the herbs are classified into that particular category.

Generalizations explains what all these herbs have in common, this will help one correlate and remember herbs in that category. However, one must be aware that nothing is absolute and that there are always exceptions.

The symptomatology section explains in general the conditions of which the category deals with. Contraindication and pharmacological action are listed at the end of the introduction.

The charts, on the other hand, are laid out across two pages. One will find it useful at the top where it gives the name of the category, it also gives the major action. This major action means that every herb listed in that category shares this common function. It is by this that the herbs are classified together into that category, therefore it is understood and not repeated again under the secondary actions.

Across the columns one will see the pharmaceutical and Chinese pin yin names, taste and energetic properties, channels entered, special comments, secondary actions, sample conditions, and dosages listed for each herb in a precise and uncluttered manner.

The secondary action does not denote a lesser degree of importance but rather in this case, it is the additional functions of each herbs beside their common function.

Many students for the purpose of test taking profess to have hard time memorizing the taste, energetic property and channels entered. It is actually very simple. One should study the section introducing the definition of taste, energy and channels entered and make correlation with the action of each herb. For example, the taste pungent in Chinese medicine has the function to disperse. This may be coupled with a warm energy which facilitates movement and relaxes the body and dispels cold. Now take an example of the herb Herba Ephedrae which is a diaphoretic warming herb that has the major action of promoting diaphoresis (sweating) and dispersing Wind cold.

One can readily see the connection between the warm and pungent qualities of the herb with its action. Because Wind cold is an external pathogenic factor that attacks first the surface of the body, we can then deduce that it will affect the lungs which is responsible for Wei Qi (the body's defensive energy). It will probably also affect the Tai Yang Channel which according to theory of disease progression, is the first stage of disease progression. The Tai Yang channel includes the Urinary Bladder channel. This is why that with an external condition, one may also have swelling usually in the face to denote the involvement with the water metabolism of the Bladder. We have just put together a system of correlation and logic without having to really memorize each of the component aspects of herbs.

The students of Chinese Herbology must always keep in mind that each of these herbs are rarely used just by itself, but rather, it is used in prescription or formulas that contain two or more herbs put together synergistically and harmoniously in such a way that encompasses the whole being. It is adaptive in that it can be changed according to the changing needs of the body.

Chinese herbal formulas and prescription writing is much more involved and is not within the scope of this book.

TABLE OF ABBREVIATIONS

abd.	abdomen
B.F.	body fluids
B.M.	bowel movement
cond.	condition
contra	contraindicated
Cx	cortex
Def.	Deficiency
diff.	difficulty
dys.	dysentery
epig.	epigastric
esp.	especially
EXT/ext	external
Fl	flos
Fo	folium
Fr	fructus
GB	Gall bladder
Hb	herba
Ht	Heart
inflam.	inflammation
ingred.	ingredient
INT/int	internal
intest.	intestinal
irreg.	irregular
KID	Kidney
LI	Large Intestine
LIV	Liver
LJ	Lower Jiao (Heater)
LU	Lungs
MJ	Middle Jiao (Heater)
obstr.	obstruction
P	Pericardium
Peri	periostracum
reten.	retention
Rm	ramulus
Rx	radix
Rz	rizoma
sem.	seminal
SI	Small Intestine
SJ	Sanjiao (Tripple Heater)
Sl.	slightly
Sm	semen (seed)
SP	Spleen
spont.	spontaneous
ST	Stomach
stagn.	stagnation
TB	tuberculosis
UB	Urinary Bladder
UJ	Upper Jiao
UTI	urinary track infection
vit.	vitamin

CHAPTER 1

DIAPHORETIC HERBS

"When [the pathogen is] lodged at the skin, induce sweat to expel it."
- Nei Jing

DEFINITION: Any herb that has the function of dispersing and expelling pathogens from the surface of the body by means of sweating is considered to be a diaphoretic herb.

GENERALIZATION: Diaphoretic herbs usually are <u>pungent</u> and act on the <u>Lung channel</u>. They all have the action to Induce sweating and Expel pathogens from the surface of the body. They are generally contraindicated in conditions of profuse sweat due to Yang Deficiency, night sweat due to Yin Deficiency, dehydration and bleeding.

SECONDARY ACTIONS:
1) Reduce swelling - through perspiration and urination.
2) Relieve measles - by inducing measle eruption (detoxification)
3) Relieve cough and asthma - by Dispersing Qi and Ventilating Lungs.
4) Stop pain (muscle ache, arthritic pains, etc.) - by Dispersing Qi stagnation.

CAUTION AND CONTRAINDICATIONS: Some herbs may have stronger diaphoretic action, thus be cautious not to induce too much perspiration to avoid damaging Yang Qi and body fluids. They are generally not recommended for profuse sweat due to Yang Deficiency, night sweat due to Yin Deficiency, bleeding and dehydration conditions.

SECTION 1

<u>DIAPHORETIC WARMING HERBS</u>

DEFINITION: Any herb that has a function of dispelling Wind Cold from the Surface of the body by means of sweating falls into this category.

GENERALIZATION: These herbs tend to be <u>pungent</u> and <u>warming</u> (to counteract the Wind and Cold factors), and have the action to Induce sweating and disperse Wind Cold.

SYMPTOMATOLOGY: The variations of Wind Cold are presented in table 1 below.

TABLE 1 - WIND COLD DIFFERENTIATION

CONDITION	ETIOLOGY	SIGNS & SYMPTOMS	PATHOLOGY
WIND COLD	Wind & Cold	severe chills with mild fever	struggle between Wei Qi (defense) & pathogens
		no sweat	Cold constrict pores
		body ache/stiff neck, headache	Wind obst. Qi flow
		P-floating, tense	pathogen at surface, Cold constricts
		T-pink, thin white coat	pathogen haven't affected inner body
*Can be complicated by:		cough or asthma	Wind Cold obst. Lung Qi, Qi can't descend
		clear/white sputum	Cold stagnates fluid
		edema-upper body	Wind Cold obst. Yang Qi
		arthritic pain & spasms	Wind Cold Attacking joints, obst. channels and collaterals
DEF. WIND COLD	Wind, Cold & Wei Qi Def.	fever & chills	struggle between Wei Qi (defense) & pathogens
		spontaneous sweat	weak Wei Qi, can't close pores
		general weakness	person is deficient
		pale face	Qi Def., and Cold
		short-of-breath	Qi Def.
		P-floating, slow and weak	weak Qi circulation
		T-pale, thin white coat	Qi Def., no supply to blood to tongue

CAUTION AND CONTRAINDICATIONS: These herbs are not appropriate for patients with spontaneous sweat, Yin and body fluid Deficiency conditions. In addition, Diaphoretic herbs should not be cooked for over 15 minutes or else the diaphoretic effects will be drastically diminished.

PHARMACOLOGICAL ACTIONS: Most of these herbs have been found to have effects of dilatation on peripheral arteries, increase capillary circulation, stimulate sweat glands, antibacterial, and antiviral, stimulate CNS regulatory functions, and analgesic effects.

16

SECTION 2

DIAPHORETIC COOLING HERBS

DEFINITION: Any herb that has the function to dispel Wind Heat from the Surface of the body by means of sweating and cooling falls into this category.

GENERALIZATION: These herbs are mostly pungent and cooling in nature, and have the common action of Dispersing Wind Heat.

SYMPTOMATOLOGY: The symptomatology of Wind Heat are presented in table 2 below.

TABLE 2 - WIND HEAT DIFFERENTIATION

CONDITION	ETIOLOGY	SIGNS & SYMPTOMS	PATHOLOGY
WIND HEAT	Wind & Heat	high fever with mild chills	struggle between Wei Qi (defense) & pathogens
		sweat	heat force fluid out
		thirst & yellow sputum	heat dry up fluid to more concentrated
		headache	Wind obst. Qi flow
		sore throat	Heat injures passage of Lungs
		P-floating, rapid	pathogen at surface, Heat facilitates
		T-pink, thin yellow coat	Heat travels faster into the body
*May be complicated by:		measles conjunctivitis other infectious disease	Toxic Heat with Wind Heat rise to eyes get into body by means of Wind

CAUTION AND CONTRAINDICATIONS: Do not boil these herbs too long for the reason that it may destroy the herb's Dispersing property (by destroying the volatile oils responsible for the diaphoretic function.) Boil for only 5-10 minutes.

PHARMACOLOGICAL ACTIONS: Most herbs in this subcategory have been found to have antibacterial, antiviral, antipyretic and analgesic actions.

pharmaceutical name	pin-yin	taste & energy	meridians	comments
Rx Angelicae Dihuerica	Bai Zhi 白芷	pungent warm	LU, ST	
Allium Fistulosum	Chong Bai 葱白	"	"	
Hb Elsholtziae	Xiang Ru 香薷	"	"	
Fl Magnolia	Xin Yi 辛夷	"	"	overdose causes dizzy & red eyes
Rz Zingiberis (fresh)	Sheng Jiang 生姜	"	"	
Fo Perillae	Zi Su 紫蘇	"	"	
Hb Asari	Xi Xin 細辛	"	LU, KID	contra. Yin Def. Heat causing head-ache, LU Heat cough
Rx et Rz Ligustici	Gao Ben 藁本	"	UB	
Hb Ledebourelliae	Fang Feng 防風	pungent sl warm sweet	UB, LIV SP	contra. Yin Def. Heat
Rm Cinnamomi	Gui Zhi 桂枝	pungent warm sweet	UB, LU HT	contra. Yin Def. Heat, Blood Heat, pregnancy
Fr Xanthii	Chong Er Zi 蒼耳子	pungent warm bitter toxic	LU	

CATEGORY: DIAPHORETIC WARMING HERBS

MAJOR ACTIONS: PROMOTE DIAPHORESIS, DISPERSE WIND COLD

secondary actions	symptoms/conditions	dose (g)
1. Remove pus, Reduce swelling 2. Relieve pain	1. skin lesion 2. Yang-Ming headache	3-10
1. Invigorate Yang Qi	1. Cold Stagn. in chest & abd. causing pain	"
1. Resolve Damp 2. Promote diuresis	1. Summer Heat & Damp 2. edema	"
1. Clear nasal passageway	1. nasal congestion, rhinorrhea	"
1. Warm LU, Relieve cough 2. Warm up Middle Jiao 3. Antidotal-sea food poison	1. LU Cold cough 2. ST Cold vomiting 3. sea food poisoning	"
1. Harmonize Middle Jiao 2. Invigorate Qi flow 3. Antidotal-sea food poison	1. vomiting 2. epig./abd. distention 3. sea food poisoning	"
1. Dispel Internal Cold 2. Warm LU 3. Relieve pain	1. Internal Cold 2. fluid retention in LU 3. headache, toothache	"
1. Dispel Wind Damp 2. Relieve pain	1. Bi syndrome 2. hernial pain	"
1. Dispel Wind Damp 2. Calm Internal Wind	1. Bi syndrome 2. Internal Wind- convulsion	"
1. Warm Channels 2. Invigorate Yang Qi	1. Bi syndrome 2. HT Yang Def. 3. Def. Wind Cold	"
1. Clear nasal passageway 2. Dispel Wind Damp 3. Relieve pain	1. nasal congestion, rhinorrhea 2. Bi syndrome 3. arthritic pain	"

CATEGORY: DIAPHORETIC—WARMING (CONT)				
pharmaceutical name	pin-yin	taste & energy	meridians	comments
Hb Ephedrae	Ma Huang 麻黄	pungent warm bitter	LU, UB	contra. in high B.P.,insomnia, excessive sweating
Hb Schizonepetae	Jing Jie 荆芥	pungent neutral	LIV, LU	
Rx et Rz Notopterygii	Qiang Huo 羌活	pungent warm bitter	UB, KID	contra. Yin Def.— headache, Def. Bi syndrome

CATEGORY: DIAPHORETIC COOLING HERBS				
pharmaceutical name	pin-yin	taste & energy	meridians	comments
Hb Mentha	Bo He 薄荷	pungent cool	LU, LIV	don't overcook
Peri Cicadae	Chan Tui 蟬蛻	sweet cold	"	
Fl Chrysanthemi	Ju Hua 菊花	pungent sweet bitter cold	"	
Hb Equisetii	Mu Zei 木賊	sweet bitter neutral	"	
Fo Mori	Sang Ye 桑葉	bitter sweet cold	"	
Fr Viticis	Man Jing Zi 蔓荆子	pungent bitter neutral	UB, LIV ST	

20

MAJOR ACTIONS: **PROMOTE DIAPHORESIS, DISPERSE WIND COLD**

secondary actions	symptoms/conditions	dose (g)
1.Ventilate LU, Relieve dyspnea 2.Promote diuresis	1.cough, dyspnea 2.acute edema (Yang) 3.Wind Cold Excess	3-10
1.Hemostatic (charred)	1.hemafecia, epitaxis	"
1.Dispel Wind Damp 2.Relieve pain	1.Bi syndrome 2.arthritic pain	"

MAJOR ACTIONS: **PROMOTE DIAPHORESIS, DISPERSE WIND HEAT**

secondary actions	symptoms/conditions	dose (g)
1.Clear head, Benefit eyes 2.Induce measle eruption	1.headache, eye inflam. 2.measles	6-30
1.Induce measle eruption 2.Brighten eyes 3.Calm endogenous Wind	1.measles 2.eye inflam. & red 3.tetany, convulsion	3-9
1.Soothe LIV, Brighten eyes	1.eye inflam. & red	6-15
1.Brighten eyes	1.blurry vision, conjunctivitis	3-12
1.Clear LIV, Brighten eyes 2.Cool blood, Stop bleeding	1.LIV Fire, red eyes 2.hemoptysis, epistaxis	3-15
1.Clear head, Brighten eyes 2.Dispel Wind Damp	1.headache, red eyes conjunctivitis 2.arthritis, Bi cond.	"

CATEGORY: DIAPHORETIC—COOLING (CONT)				
pharmaceutical name	pin-yin	taste & energy	meridians	comments
Rx Puerariae	Ge Gen 葛根	Pungent sweet cold	SP, ST UB	
Rz Cimicifugae	Sheng Ma 升麻	pungent sweet sl.cold	LU, L.I. ST, SP	
Rx Bupleuri	Chai Hu 柴胡	pungent bitter cool	LIV, P SJ, GB	
Fr Arctii	Niu Bang Zi 牛蒡子	pungent bitter cold	LU, ST	
Sm Sojae Preparatae	Dan Dou Chi 淡豆豉	pungent sweet bitter cold	"	
Fl Chrysanthemi Indicum	Ye Ju Hua 野菊花	bitter neutral	SP, HT LIV, KID	
Hb Lamnae	Fu Ping 浮萍	pungent cold	LU	caution: def. cond, spontaneous sweat

secondary actions	symptoms/conditions	dose (g)
1.Relieve muscle aches 2.Clear Heat, Quench thirst 3.Raise Spleen Yang 4.Induce measle eruption	1.stiff neck & shoulder 2.thirst, dehydration 3.chronic diarrhea 4.measles	"
1.Clear Toxic Heat 2.Raise Yang Qi 3.Induce measle eruption	1.skin lesions 2.organ prolapse 3.measles	"
1.Soothe LIV, Remove Stagnant Qi 2.Raise Yang Qi	1.LIV Qi Stagnation 2.organ prolapse	"
1.Induce measle eruption 2.Clear Toxic Heat 3.Benefit the throat	1.measles 2.skin lesions 3.sore throat	"
1.Relieve restlessness	1.restlessness, fidgety	"
1.Clear Heat & Toxin 2.Lower blood pressure	1.skin lesions, sore throat 2.high blood pressure	"
1.Promote Diuresis, Reduce swelling	1.measles, Wind Damp Bi 2.edema, dysuria	3-6

CHAPTER 2

ANTIPYRETIC/HEAT CLEARING HERBS

DEFINITION: Any herb that has the function of Clearing Heat and Purging Fire from the Interior of the body is considered to be an antipyretic herb.

GENERALIZATION: Antipyretic herbs are mostly cold or cooling in nature, bitter in taste, and often enter the channels corresponding to their action. They all have the action to Clear Heat or Purge Fire depending on the potency of the individual herb. Below in the differentiation section are tables showing various heat conditions through differentiation according to Chinese Medical theories.

DIFFERENTIATION: Table 3 and 4 are differentiations of Heat conditions through two theoretical models. These are utilized to demonstrate the location of the pathogen and the relative strength of both the pathogenic factor, the Heat, and the Antipathogenic factor, the body.

TABLE 3 - EIGHT PRINCIPLES DIFFERENTIATION OF HEAT

LOCATION OF PATHOGEN	SIGNS & SYMPTOMS
EXTERNAL HEAT	high fever & mild chills, sweat, thirst headache, sore throat, yellow sputum, P-floating and rapid, T-pink, slightly yellow coat
INTERNAL HEAT	high fever without chills, thirst, constipation, concentrated urine, fear of heat, irritability, sweat, P-rapid, T-red, yellow coat
CHARACTER. CONDITION	SIGNS & SYMPTOMS
EXCESS HEAT	red face and eyes, high fever, excess thirst, excess sweat, constipation, scanty & concentrated urine, bitter taste in mouth, mania, irritability, foul breath, delirium, P-rapid, full, T-red, yellow dry coat
DEFICIENT HEAT (Yin Deficiency - or False Heat)	low afternoon fever, irritability, night sweats, flushed cheeks, insomnia, feverish palms, soles and chest, dry mouth, P-rapid & thready, T-red, little or no coat

TABLE 4: WEI, QI, YING AND XUE DIFFERENTIATION
(Stages of febrile disease progression)

CONDITION	SIGNS & SYMPTOMS	PATHOLOGY
WEI level	High fever & mild chills sweat, thirst, headache, sore throat, yellow sputum, P-floating and rapid, T-pink slightly yellow coat	attack of Heat, Dryness & Summer Heat to Exterior of the body
QI level	high fever, no chills, irritability, excess sweat, excess thirst, constipation, abdominal pain, red face, fear of heat, cough, yellow sputum, concentrated urine, P-full, stong and flooding, T-red with yellow coat	the pathogens attack through the surface and are now on the Interior of the body most likely affect the Lungs, Stomach or Large Intestine
YING level	fever, especially late afternoons and evenings, insomnia, irritability, occasional delirium, skin petechiaes, P-rapid and thready, T-dry and scarlet red	now the Heat further penetrates to deeper body, most likely to affect the Pericardium and disturbs the spirit
XUE level	high fever, delirium, insomnia, mania, coma, signs of bleeding, i.e.vomiting of blood, nose bleed, bloody stool, bruising underneath the skin etc. or tremors & spasms, P-rapid and thready, T-dark red with prickles, brown burnt coat	the pathogenic Heat at the deepest level is driving blood out of vessels & invade the Heart (spirit), starting to create a current (LIV Wind)

Due to its dynamic Yang characteristics, the Heat pathogen has a wide spread effect on the body in disease conditions. To fully encompass the diversity of the pathological conditions, Antipyretic herbs are further divided into subcategories, and they are listed below.

FIVE TYPES OF ANTYPRETIC HERBS:

1. HEAT CLEARING & FIRE PURGING HERBS
   A. HERBS THAT CLEAR HEAT IN THE "QI" STAGE

B. HERBS THAT CLEAR HEAT & DRY UP DAMPNESS

2. <u>HEAT CLEARING & BLOOD COOLING HERBS</u>

3. <u>FALSE HEAT CLEARING (YIN DEFICIENT HEAT) HERBS</u>

4. <u>HEAT CLEARING & ANTI-TOXIN HERBS</u>
   A. HERBS FOR FEBRILE DISEASE
   B. HERBS FOR TOXIC SKIN LESIONS
   C. HERBS FOR TOXIC DYSENTERY
   D. HERBS FOR THROAT INFLAMMATION

5. <u>HEAT CLEARING & EYES BRIGHTENING HERBS</u>

CAUTIONS AND CONTRAINDICATIONS: These herbs should not be used for Cold or Yang Deficiency conditions.

PHARMACOLOGICAL ACTIONS: Recent studies found these herbs to have highly potent antipyretic (reduce fever) action. Some are antibacterial and anti-viral and are effective for infectious diseases such as meningitis, bronchitis, and etc. Herbs such as Blood Cooling herbs also have antihypertensive and mild hemostatic functions. And many also posses diuretic, antifungal, and anti-inflammatory functions.

SECTION 1

HEAT CLEARING & FIRE PURGING HERBS

A. HERBS THAT CLEAR HEAT IN THE "QI" STAGE

DEFINITION: Any herb that has the function of clearing and expelling pathogenic Heat from the Qi level of the body.

GENERALIZATION: These herbs tend to be <u>bitter</u>, <u>sweet</u> and <u>cold</u>, and mainly act on the <u>Lung</u>, <u>Stomach</u> and a few other channels. They are likely to damage the Spleen and Stomach because of their bitter and cold nature, thus, when the condition is complicated with Spleen & Stomach weakness, the addition of Spleen and Stomach tonics is recommended.

SYMPTOMATOLOGY: High fever, no chills, irritability, excess sweat, excess thirst, constipation, abdominal pain, red face, fear of heat, cough, yellow sputum, concentrated urine, pulse is full, strong and flooding, tongue is red with yellow coating.

CAUTION AND CONTRAINDICATIONS: It is not recommended for Spleen and Stomach weakness and cold condition.

B. HERBS THAT CLEAR HEAT AND DRY UP DAMPNESS

DEFINITION: Any herb that has the major action of dispelling Heat and Dampness from the body is considered to be a Damp Heat Resolving herb.

GENERALIZATION: Damp Heat Resolving herbs generally are bitter and cold, they will easily injure the Spleen and Stomach if used excessively. Therefore, exercise caution when using them in Spleen and Stomach Deficiency conditions, as not to further weaken these organs. When necessary, one should combine Spleen and Stomach Tonics with the prescription.

SYMPTOMATOLOGY: Fullness & distension in chest, dysentery, diarrhea, dysuria with concentrated urine, eczema, leukorrhea, jaundice, lack of appetite, heaviness sensation, high fever or constant low fever, tongue is yellow with greasy coating, pulse is rapid and slippery.

CAUTIONS AND CONTRAINDICATIONS: It is not recommended for Spleen and Stomach weakness and Cold.

SECTION 2

HEAT CLEARING & BLOOD COOLING HERBS

DEFINITION: Any herb that helps to dispel Excess Heat from the Blood stage is considered a Blood Heat Clearing herb.

GENERALIZATION: These herbs are cold or cooling in nature, they are used in conditions of Excess Heat in the Ying or Xue (blood) stage of Febrile Disease and also Yin Def. Heat. Some herbs also have hemostatic action. Also, when pathogenic Heat enters the Yin part of the body (Ying and blood level) the body's Yin and fluids are dried up, therefore, some of the herbs also nourish the Yin.

SYMPTOMATOLOGY: Classical Chinese Medicine observed that febrile diseases progress through various stages. A theoretical model was to developed to map out these stages. It was called the Wei, Qi, Ying and Xue Differentiation. In this particular section, Heat Clearing & Blood Cooling herbs deals mainly with Heat conditions in the last two stages of its progression. (Please refer to table 4 for information on the two preceding stages) Below is table 5 listing the symptomatology of Heat of the Ying and Xue stages.

27

TABLE 5 – HEAT OF THE YING AND THE XUE STAGES

CONDITION	SIGNS & SYMPTOMS	PATHOLOGY
Heat in the Ying stage	fever, especially late afternoons and evenings, insomnia irritability, occasional delirium, skin petechiaes, P-rapid and thready, T-dry and scarlet red	now the Heat further penetrates to deeper body, most likely to affect the Pericardium and disturbs the spirit
Heat in the Xue stage (blood)	high fever, delirium, insomnia, mania, coma, signs of bleeding, i.g.vomiting of blood, nose bleed, bloody stool, bruising underneath the skin, etc, or tremors & spasms, P-rapid and thready, T-dark red with prickles, brown burnt coat	pathogenic Heat at the deepest level is driving blood out of vessels & invade the heart (spirit), starting to create a current (LIV Wind)

SECTION 3:

FALSE HEAT CLEARING (YIN DEFICIENT HEAT CLEARING) HERBS

DEFINITION: Any herb that has the major action of cooling Heat arising from insufficiency of Yin which is of deficient nature and not a "Real" excess Heat, also referred to as False Heat, is regard as a False Heat Clearing herb.

GENERALIZATION: These herbs are often used in False Heat conditions in the late stage of febrile diseases, chronic degenerative diseases and Yin Deficiency conditions. Make sure that one takes care of the underlying Yin Deficiency condition by combining with Yin Tonic herbs in the prescription.

SYMPTOMATOLOGY: Low afternoon fever, irritability, night sweat, flushed cheeks, insomnia, feverish palms, soles and chest, dry mouth and throat especially at night, in severe cases one may experience "bone steaming" sensa- tion as if the heat were evaporating from the bones, pulse is rapid and thready, tongue is red with little or no coating.

SECTION 4

HEAT CLEARING AND ANTITOXIN HERBS

DEFINITION: Herbs in this category have actions that cover a broad spectrum of conditions, but mainly infections such as various febrile diseases i.e. mumps, encephalitis, bacterial dysentery, skin lesions such as eriseplis, boils, furuncles, abscesses, and throat disorders such as strep. throat, diptheria and tonsillitis, etc.. Some also counteract snake poisoning, therefore achieving its action of Clear Heat and Detoxify.

A. HERBS FOR FEBRILE DISEASE

DEFINITION: Herbs in this subcategory are used to treat febrile diseases mainly in the Wei and Qi stage. Although they are also useful in the later stages when combined properly with herbs from other subcategories of Antipy-retic Herbs.

GENERALIZATION: These herbs are mostly bitter and cooling. Generally they are used for infections and early stages of febrile disease, frequently combined with Diaphoretic herbs, and Internal Toxic Heat conditions that have progressed from the Exterior of the body.

SYMPTOMATOLOGY: high fever, sore throat, irritability, swollen, red and painful lymph glands, cough with yellow sputum, red face, scanty concen-trated urine, suppurative skin lesions, tongue is red with yellow coating, pulse is rapid, full and/or floating.

B. HERBS FOR TOXIC SKIN LESIONS

DEFINITION: Any herb that helps to dispel Heat and Toxin and aids healing suppurative skin lesions is considered a Skin Toxin Clearing Herb.

GENERALIZATION: Herbs in this subcategory are mostly bitter and cold. They are effective in combating skin lesions that result from infections by bacteria, virus, fungus and acute inflammatory stage of a skin condition. Most frequently, there will be suppuration or discharge from the lesions which is further indicative of the toxicity. These herb are used externally as well.

SYMPTOMATOLOGY: Toxic Heat in the body may cause skin lesions or sores that are red, hot, swollen, and painful. Some have pus or other foul discharge from the lesion. Accompanying the skin lesion, one may have fever and burning and painful urination.

SAMPLE SKIN DISEASES: boils, carbuncles, furuncles, abscesses (including that affecting the organs), ulcerations, mastitis, eriseplis, herpes zoster, herpes genitalia, eczema, etc.

C. HERBS FOR TOXIC DYSENTERY

DEFINITION: Any herbs that has the major action of dispelling toxins from "Toxic" Dysentery condition, thus relieving the dysentery, is considered a Dysentery Clearing Herb.

GENERALIZATION: The herbs in this category are used mainly in dysentery conditions caused by bacteria and parasites that are introduced through unsanitary diet. The term "Toxic" in Chinese Medicine often denotes an infection from micro-organisms.

SYMPTOMATOLOGY: Signs and symptoms often include acute diarrhea with tenesmus, abdominal pain, foul smelling stools accompanied by pus or blood, fever and fatigue.

SAMPLE CONDITIONS: bacillary dysentery, food poisoning, amoebic dysentery, cholera, etc..

D. HERBS FOR THROAT INFLAMMATION

DEFINITION: Any herb that helps dispel Toxins and Heat from the throat, thus soothing the irritations in the throat, falls under this category.

GENERALIZATION: These herbs are mostly bitter and cold, and enter the Lung channel. They are mainly used in throat infections and can be used internally and also in powder form to be sprayed directly to soothe the throat.

SYMPTOMATOLOGY: One may experience sore throat, swollen lymph glands around the throat, dryness in the throat, hoarseness or loss of voice, fever, and inability to swallow.

SAMPLE CONDITIONS: tonsillitis, sore throat due to influenza, streptococcus or staphylococcus infection, diphtheria, Vincent's Angina, infectious mononucleosis, etc.

SECTION 5

HEAT CLEARING & EYE BRIGHTENING HERBS

DEFINITION: Any herb that has the function to clear Heat from the eyes, thus alleviating acute eye distress, falls under this category.

GENERALIZATION: These herbs are generally sweet, bitter and cooling in nature. They all enter the liver channel. Because acute eye disorders are commonly due to either External Wind Heat or Liver Heat Rising, Diaphoretic herbs, Liver heat Clearing herbs and Liver & Kidney tonics, should be combined appropriately. Sometimes, these herbs can be boiled to externally "steam" the eyes or stuffed into a pillow as an external application. Some also have the action of lowering the blood pressure.

SYMPTOMATOLOGY: Heat tend to rise in nature so it easily affects the upper part of the body especially the eyes causing various eye disorders. Below in table 6, it shows the various types of Heat conditions that causes eye disorder.

TABLE 6 – DIFFERENTIATION OF EYE DISORDERS

CONDITION	SIGNS & SYMPTOMS
WIND HEAT	redness, painful, and swollen eye with heat sensation, yellowish, pus discharge with other symptoms of Wind Heat condition
EXCESS LIVER	redness, painful, swollen eye, red face easily angered, dryness of the eye, headache vertigo, tinnitus, dry throat, P-rapid and full, T-red with yellow coat
DEF. LIVER HEAT (Liver Yin Def.)	red, achy and dry eye, flushed cheeks dizziness, tinnitus, blurry vision irritability, insomnia, night sweat, heat sensation in the palms, soles and chest area P-rapid and thready, T-red, thin or no coat

CAUTIONS AND CONTRAINDICATIONS: Many of these herbs possess lubricating function, thus use with caution in diarrhea cases.

CATEGORY: HEAT CLEARING & FIRE PURGING HERBS

pharmaceutical name	pin-yin	taste & energy	meridians	comments
Plumula Nelumbinis	Lian Zi Xin 蓮子心	bitter cold	HT	
Fr Gardenia	Zhi Zi 栀子	"	HT, LIV ST, SJ	
Fel Ursi	Xiong Dan 熊胆	"	LIV, HT GB	
Rz Anemarrhenae	Zhi Mu 知母	bitter sweet cold	LU, ST KID	contra. for person with diarrhea
Hb Lophatheri	Dan Zhu Ye 淡竹葉	sweet cold bland	HT, ST SI	
Gypsum Fibrosum	Shi Gao 石膏	pungent sweet	LU, ST	
Calcitum	Han Shui Shi 寒水石	salty cold	ST, KID	
Citrullus Vulgaris Shrad	Xi Gua 西瓜	sweet bland cold	HT, SP	
Fo Nelumbinis	He Ye 荷葉	bitter neutrl	SP, ST	

CATEGORY: HERBS THAT CLEAR HEAT & DRY DAMPNESS

pharmaceutical name	pin-yin	taste & energy	meridians	comments
Rx Gentianae	Long Dan Cao 龍胆草	bitter cold	LIV, GB ST	

MAJOR ACTIONS: CLEAR HEAT IN THE QI STAGE

secondary actions	symptoms/conditions	dose (g)
1.Clear Heart Fire	1.Heart Fire 2.hypertension	1.5-6
1.Clear Heat and Damp 2.Cool Blood 3.Relieve restlessness	1.LIV Fire 2.Damp Heat jaundice 3.LIV Blood Heat	3-10
1.Clear LIV Heat 2.Anti-helmenthic 3.Relieve Yang Jaundice	1.jaundice 2.intestinal worms	0.1-0.3
1.Nourish Yin 2.Moisten Dryness	1.Yin Deficiency Heat	6-12
1.Ease urination 2.Relieve restlessness	1.dysuria 2.irritability 3.fidgety	10-15
1.Nourish Body Fluids 2.EXT-Arrest wounds	1.LU or ST Heat 2.non-healing wounds	15-60
1.Clear Heart Fire 2.Aid wound healing	1.Heat in Qi Stage 2.burns, erisepelas	9-30
1.Ease urination 2.Relieve restlessness	1.dysuria 2.fidgety 3.thirst	12-60
1.Clear Summer Heat 2.Raise Pure Yang	1.Summer Heat	use 1/4 leaf

MAJOR ACTIONS: CLEAR HEAT, DRY DAMP

secondary actions	symptoms/conditions	dose (g)
1.Purge LIV Fire	1.Excess LIV Fire 2.LIV Wind	3-6

pharmaceutical name	pin-yin	taste & energy	meridians	comments
Rx Scutellariae	Huang Qin 黄芩	"	LU, LIV GB, ST LI	
Rx Sophorae Flavescentis	Gu Shen 苦参	"	HT, LIV ST, UB LI	contra. with Rx Veratri
Cx Phellodendri	Huang Bai 黄柏	"	KID, UB LI	
Rz Coptidis	Huang Lian 黄连	"	HT, LIV ST, LI	
Sm Dolichoris	Bai Bian Dou 白扁豆	sweet warm	SP, ST	
Sm Sojae Germinatum	Da Dou Huang Xiang 大豆黄卷	sweet neutral	ST	

CATEGORY: HEAT DISPELLING, BLOOD COOLING HERBS				
pharmaceutical name	pin-yin	taste & energy	meridians	comments
Rx Rehmanniae (raw)	Sheng Di Huang 生地黄	sweet bitter cold	HT, LIV KID	
Rx Scrophulariae	Xuan Shen 玄参	sweet bitter salty cold	LU, ST KID	conta. with Rx Veratri
Cx Moutan Radicis	Mu Dan Pi 牡丹皮	bitter pungent sl.cold	HT, LIV KID	contra. pregnancy
Rx Macrotomiae seu Lithospermi	Zi Cao 紫草	sweet cold	HT, LIV	
Cornu Bubali	Shui Niu Jiao 水牛角	bitter, salty, cold	Liv., Ht., St	

34

secondary actions	symptoms/conditions	dose (g)
1.Detoxify 2.Hemostatic 3.Stabalize fetus	1.skin disease 2.Blood Heat bleeding 3.fetal hypermotility	3-10
1.Dispel Wind 2.Anti-helminthic 3.Ease urination	1.itching 2.fungal infections 3.Damp Heat dysuria	3-10
1.Clear Toxic Heat 2.Clear Yin Deficiency Heat	1.skin disease 2.Yin Deficiency Heat	3-10
1.Clear Heat 2.Detoxify	1.bleeding conditions 2.ST and HT Fire	1-5
1.Clear Summer Heat 2.Tonify SP, Resolve Damp 3.Detoxify	1.Summer Heat & Damp 2.sea food poisoning	3-12
1.Clear Heat 2.Resolve Damp	1.Summer Heat 2.Damp, edema 3.Bi syndrome	3-15

MAJOR ACTIONS: DISPELL HEAT, COOL BLOOD

secondary actions	symptoms/conditions	dose (g)
1.Nourish Yin 2.Nourish Body Fluids	1.Yin Deficiency Heat	9-30
1.Nourish Yin 2.Detoxify 3.Dissolve Hardenings	1.LU Yin Deficiency 2.scrofula	9-30
1.Invigorate Blood flow 2.Remove Stagnation	1.amenorrhea 2.dysmenorrhea 3.tumors	6-12
1.Detoxify 2.Induce measle eruption	1.skin diseases 2.measles 3.B.F. Def.constipation	3-10
1.Clears Heat, Detox. 2.Cools blood, Stops bleeding	1.Excess Heat, Blood Heat 2.High Fever, delirium 3.bleeding, convulsion	30-120g

pharmaceutical name	pin-yin	taste & energy	meridians	comments
Rz Immperatae	Bai Mao Gen 白茅根	"	LU, ST SI, UB	
Cornu Rhinoceri Asiatica	Xi Jiao 犀角	salty cold	HT, LIV ST	contra. pregnancy. Use in powder form.

CATEGORY: FALSE HEAT CLEARING HERBS

pharmaceutical name	pin-yin	taste & energy	meridians	commments
Hb Artemisiae Chinghao	Qing Hao 青蒿	"	LIV, GB UB	don't overcook
Cx Lycii Radicis	Di Gu Pi 地骨皮	sweet bland cold	LU, KID	
Rx Cynanchi Atrati	Bai Wei 白薇	bitter salty cold	LIV, KID ST	
Rx Stellariae Dichotomae	Ying Chai Hu 銀柴胡	sweet sl.cold	LIV, ST	

CATEGORY: HEAT CLEARING & ANTITOXIN HERBS

pharmaceutical name	pin-yin	taste & energy	meridians	comments
Rx Pulsatillae	Bai Tou Weng 白頭翁	bitter cold	LI	
Cx Dictamni Radicus	Bai Xian Pi 白蘚皮	"	SP, ST	
Fr Forsythiae	Lian Qiao 連翹	"	HT, LU GB	

36

1.Cool Blood to stop bleeding 2.Promote Diuresis	1.epistaxis, hematuria, hematemesis 2.edema, dysuria, jaundice	9–30 fresh–use 30–60
1.Clear HT, Calm Spirit 2.Clear Toxic Heat 3.Hemostatic	1.Ying/Xue Stage Heat 2.Blood Heat bleeding	1.5–6

MAJOR ACTIONS: CLEAR FALSE HEAT (YIN DEF. HEAT)

secondary actions	symptoms/conditions	dose (g)
1.Anti–malaria (king herb) 2.Clear Deficiency Heat	1.malaria 2.Yin Deficiency Heat	3–9
1.Clear LU Heat 2.Clear Deficiency Heat	1.LU Heat cough 2.Yin Deficiency Heat 3.hypertension	6–12
1.Clear Deficiency Heat 2.Ease urination 3.Detoxify	1.Deficiency Heat 2.urinary problems 3.skin disease	3–9
1.Clear Deficiency Heat 2.Clear malnutrition fever	1.Yin Deficiency Heat 2.malnutrition fever	3–10

MAJOR ACTIONS: CLEAR HEAT, DETOXIFY

secondary actions	symptoms/conditions	dose (g)
1.Cool Blood 2.Stop dysentery	1.bloody dysentery 2.acute bacterial dys. 3.amoebic dysentery	6–15
1.Dispell Wind 2.Remove Damp	1.itchy conditions 2.Bi syndrome 3.jaundice	4–10
1.Resolve exudates 2.Soften Hardenings	1.Upper Jiao Heat 2.tuberculosis 3.scrofula	6–16

Rx Isatidis	Ban Lang Gen 板藍根	"	HT, LU	use with Fm Isatidis
Fm Isatidis	Da Qing Ye 大青葉	bitter extreme cold	HT, LU ST	use with Rx Isatidis
Fl Lonicerae	Jin Yin Hua 金銀花	sweet cold	LU, ST LI	use up to 60g in severe cases
Rz Smilacis Glabrae	Tu Fu Ling 土茯苓	sweet bland neutral	LIV, ST	
Rx Echinopiae	Lou Lu 漏蘆	bitter cold	ST	
Rx Sophorae Subprostratae	Shan Dou Gen 山豆根	"	HT, LU LI	
Hb Taraxaci	Pu Gong Ying 蒲公英	bitter sweet cold	LIV, ST	
Rx Ampelopsis	Bai Lian 白蘞	pungent bitter sl.cold	HT, LIV SP	contra. with Rx Aconiti
Rz Belamcandae	She Gan 射干	bitter cold toxic	LU, LIV	contra. pregnant

1.Cool Blood 2.Benefit throat	1.skin petechiae 2.throat inflammation	15-30
1.Cool Blood	1.severe Heat	10-16
1.Cool Blood 2.Stop dysentery	1.charred for bloody dysentery	10-16
1.Remove Damp 2.Benefit joints	1.syphilis 2.syphilitic arthritis 3.Heat Ling syndrome	15-60
1.Reduce swelling 2.Resolve Abscess 3.Promote lactation	1.breast abscess, mastitis, lactostasis	3-12
1.Counteract tumors 2.Benefit throat	1.respiratory tract cancer, UB cancer 2.gingivitis, sore throat	6-9
1.Clear Heat and Toxins in Blood 2.Resolve Damp	1.boils, furuncles mastitis, etc. 2.jaundice, hepatitis, acute UTI	10-30
1.Reduce swelling, Remove Damp 2.Resolve Abscess, Stop pain 3.Aids wound healing	1.abscess, carbuncles furuncles, burns	3-10
1.Reduce swelling 2.Benefit throat 3.Descend Qi, Expel Phlegm	1.edema of glottis 2.acute tonsilitis/ laryngitis 3.LU Heat-cough/wheezing with profuse sputum	6-9

CATEGORY: HEAT CLEARING & EYE BRIGHTENING HERBS				
pharmaceutical name	pin-yin	taste & energy	meridians	comments
Sm Cassiae Torae	Jue Ming Zi 决明子	sweet bitter salty sl.cold	LIV, LI	
Spica Prunellae	Xia Gu Cao 夏枯草	bitter pungent cold	LIV, GB	
Rz Phragmitis	Lu Gen 蘆根	sweet cold	LU, ST	
Vespertili Excrementum	Yie Min Sha 夜明砂	pungent cold	LIV	

MAJOR ACTIONS: CLEAR HEAT, BRIGHTEN EYES

secondary actions	symptoms/conditions	dose (g)
1.Brighten eyes 2.Relieve constipation	1.LIV Fire 2.constipation 3.hypertension	9-15
1.Clear LIV Fire 2.Disperse Stagnations 3.Lower blood pressure	1.LIV Fire 2.scrofula 3.hypertension	6-10
1.Nourish Body Fluids 2.Stop vomiting 3.Ease urination	1.Quenches thirst 2.ST Heat vomiting 3.LU Heat cough,dysuria	15-30
1.Soothe LIV 2.Remove Stagnation	1.red, painful, inflam. eyes, eye hemorrhage, cataracts, spots	3-9

CHAPTER 3

ANTI-MALARIAL HERBS

DEFINITION: Any herb that helps to control and inhibit malaria falls into this category.

GENERALIZATION: These herbs traditionally have been observed to be effective in the treatment of malaria. They help control the paroxysmal attacks of fever and chills. Most are bitter, pungent and cooling and some are toxic. To effectively treat malaria, one must also combine herbs according to the stages of the condition. When the condition is still exogenous, one should add diaphoretic herbs, if complicated by Summer Heat and Damp factors, one should seek to resolve and dispel these pathogens at the same time. Often times, it is necessary to strengthen and regulate Stomach and Spleen and tonify and nourish Qi and blood afterwards to prevent recurrence of the condition.

SYMPTOMATOLOGY: Malaria is an infectious disease due to the presence of protozoan parasites within the blood which are generally transmitted by mosquito. One may experience periodic alternating chills and fever, sweating, epigastric pain, diarrhea, low appetite, nausea and a coated tongue.

CAUTION AND CONTRAINDICATIONS: Some herbs are toxic. Thus exercise caution over the amount and time period of administering herbs. A few of them also have emetic actions.

PHARMACOLOGICAL ACTIONS: These herbs have been found to have antimalarial effects, some much more potent then quinine, the alkaloid used to treat malaria in modern medicine.

CATEGORY: ANTIMALARIAL HERBS				
pharmaceutical name	pin-yin	taste & energy	meridians	comments
Hb Artemisiae Chinghao	Qing Hao 青 蒿	bitter pungent cold	LIV, GB UB	don't overcook

MAJOR ACTIONS: CLEAR FALSE HEAT (YIN DEF. HEAT)		
secondary actions	symptoms/conditions	dose (g)
1.Anti-malaria (king herb) 2.Clear Deficiency Heat	1.malaria 2.Yin Deficiency Heat	3-9

CHAPTER 4

PHLEGM RESOLVING HERBS

"the spleen is the creator of phlegm and the lung is the container of phlegm."

- Classics

DEFINITION: Any herb that helps to dissolve and excrete phlegm out of the lungs and other parts of the body falls into this category.

GENERALIZATION: There are two subcategories of Phlegm Resolving herbs, mainly that of the Cold Phlegm and Heat Phlegm Resolving herbs. They each have different properties and are used to treat varied conditions. Because of the stagnant characteristic of Phlegm, it tends to obstruct and affect different parts of the body such as the Lungs, the Heart Orifice, Stomach and Spleen and Channels and Collaterals.

PHARMACOLOGICAL ACTIONS: These herbs have been found to have antimicrobial, antispasmodic and expectorant effects. Some herbs, in addition, are antineoplastic and antitussive in action.

SECTION ONE

COLD PHLEGM RESOLVING HERBS

DEFINITION: Any herb that acts to Warm up the Lungs and dispel the Cold, dry up the Dampness and dissolve the Phlegm falls into this category.

GENERALIZATION: Cold Phlegm Resolving herbs are generally <u>pungent</u>, <u>warming</u> and <u>drying</u>, and of course, they all enter the <u>Lungs</u> and <u>Spleen</u>.

SYMPTOMATOLOGY: Generally speaking, white copious mucous, white and greasy coating on the tongue and a slippery pulse are the obvious signs.
    Depending on where the phlegm affects the body it can cause different symptoms. When it obstructs the Lungs, one may have cough, dyspnea, asthma, and white phlegm; when it mists the Heart Orifice, the Spirit is disturbed, hence one may see delirium, mania, hysteria, neurosis and even unconsciousness; when it invades the Stomach and Spleen, one may see nausea, vomiting, diarrhea; it can be found lodged in the Channels and the muscles as lumps, cysts, T.B., scrofula, and numbness and even tumors.

CONTRAINDICATIONS: Some of the herbs, such as Rz Pinellia and Rz Arisaematis, are very potent and drying, therefore, refrain from use in conditions of dry cough due to Lung Yin Deficiency, Hemoptysis due to Lung Heat and severe Heat Phlegm obstructing the Lungs.

SECTION TWO

HEAT PHLEGM RESOLVING HERBS

DEFINITION: Any herb that helps to resolve Heat Phlegm in the body falls into this category.

GENERALIZATION: Herbs in this category tend to be <u>cooling</u> in nature. They all enter the <u>Lungs</u> and some have additional actions such as lubricate the Lungs, Soften Hardening, etc. Because Heat is the complicating factor in this condition, it may manifest with symptoms of dryness and Excess Heat, so sometimes Antipyretics and Yin Tonics should be supplemented to the prescription along with Phlegm Resolving herbs to take care of the problem.

SYMPTOMATOLOGY: Very similar to that found in the Cold Phlegm Resolving section except symptoms of Heat are prominent. Apparent signs are often yellow and thick sputum, not very easily coughed up, and may be accompanied by fever and thirst, sometimes hemoptysis and chest pain with cough.
   Also depending on where the Heat Phlegm affects the body, symptoms are similar and correspond to those listed in the Cold Phlegm section with addition of perhaps fever and signs of infections.

CONTRAINDICATIONS: Because some of the herbs Soften Hardening, it is contraindicated in pregnancy.

CATEGORY: COLD PHLEGM RESOLVING HERBS

pharmaceutical name	pin-yin	taste & energy	meridians	comments
Rx Platycodi	Jie Geng 桔梗	bitter pungent neutral	LU	
Sm Sinapis Alba	Ba Jie Zi 白芥子	pungent warm	"	
Spina Gleditsiae	Zao Jiao Chi 皂角刺	pungent warm sl.toxic	LU, LI	contra. pregnant, Qi Def., Yin Def., bleeding
Rz Pinelliae	Ban Xia 半夏	pungent warm toxic	SP, ST LU	prepare with Ginger or Alumen to reduce toxicity
Rz Arisaematis	Tian Nan Xing 天南星	bitter pungent warm toxic	LU, LIV SP	contra. pregnant prepare with Ginger or Alumen to reduce toxicity
Rx Aconiti Coreani	Bai Fu Zi 白附子	pungent sweet hot toxic	SP, LIV ST	contra. Yin & Blood Deficiency, and Febrile Diseases
Rz et Rx Cynanchi Stauntoni	Bai Qian 白前	pungent sweet sl.warm	LU	
Fl Inulae	Xuan Fu Hua 旋覆花	bitter pungent salty sl.warm	LU, SP ST, LI	
Peri Citri Erthrocarpae	Ju Hong 橘紅	pungent, bitter, warm	Lu, Sp	

MAJOR ACTIONS: DRY DAMPNESS, RESOLVE COLD PHLEGM

secondary actions	symptoms/conditions	dose (g)
1.Ventilate LU Qi 2.Remove Pus	1.any cough 2.lung abscess	3-9
1.Warms LU 2.Invigorate Qi 3.Disperse Hardenings	1.Cold Phlegm in LU 2.Phlegm-Damp obst. Jing-Luo 3.nodules	"
1.Clear Orifices	1.Phlegm Misting HT 2.Phlegm clogging Orifices	"
1.Descend Rebellious Qi 2.Stop vomiting 3.Disperse Hardenings	1.vomiting 2.chest fullness 3.scrofula,Plumpit sens.	5-9
1.Dispell Wind 2.Anti-convulsion	1.Wind Phlegm 2.Ext.-skin lesions 3.uterine carcinoma	" (raw - 0.3-1)
1.Dispell Wind 2.Anti-convulsion 3,Detoxify 4.Disperse Hardenings	1.Wind Phlegm 2.scrofula, T.B. 3.snake bites	3-5
1.Descend Rebellious Qi 2.Stop cough	1.cough	3-9
1.Diuretic 2.Descend Rebellious Qi 3.Stop vomiting	1.Phlegm-Damp in LU 2.vomiting, belching	"
1.Dries Dampness, Resolves Phlegm	1.Phlegm Damp cough, tenacious white phlegm	3-12g

CATEGORY: HEAT PHLEGM RESOLVING HERBS				
pharmaceutical name	pin-yin	taste & energy	meridians	comments
Pumice	Fu Hai Shi 浮海石	salty cold	LU	
Rx Peucedani	Qian Hu 前胡	bitter pungent sl.cold	"	
Bulbus Fritillariae Cirrhosae	Chuan Bei Mu 川贝母	bitter sweet sl.cold	LU, HT	contra. with Rx Aconiti
Bulbus Fritillariae Thunbergii	Zhe Bei Mu 浙贝母	bitter cold	"	contra. with Rx Aconiti
Bambusae in Taenia	Zhu Ru 竹茹	sweet sl.cold	ST, LU GB	
Rx Adenophorae	Nan Sha Shen 南沙参	"	LU, ST	action similar to Glehnia but weaker
Rx Trichosanthis	Tian Hua Fen 天花粉	bitter sl.sweet cold	"	
Fr Trichosanthis	Gua Lou 瓜蒌	sweet cold	LU, ST LI	
Sm Trichosanthis	Gua Shi Ren 瓜蒌仁	"	"	
Succus Bambusae	Zhu Li 竹沥	sweet very-cold	HT, LU ST	

MAJOR ACTIONS:	RESOLVE HEAT PHLEGM	
secondary actions	symptoms/conditions	dose (g)
1.Soften Hardenings	1.scrofula, T.B. 2.Stone Lin syndrome	6-9
1.Descend LU Qi 2.Disperse Wind Heat	1.Wind Heat cough	3-9
1.Clear Heat 2.Disperse Hardenings 3.Moisten Lungs 4.Stop cough	1.lung abscess 2.scrofula 3.LU dryness-cough	3-9
1.Clear Heat 2.Disperse Hardenings 3.Stop cough	1.lung abscess 2.scrofula 3.LU Heat cough	"
1.Relieve Restlessness 2.Stop vomiting 3.Stabilize fetus	1.GB Heat affecting HT 2.ST Heat-vomiting 3.fetal hypermotility	6-9
1.Moisten LU 2.Strengthen Qi	1.dry cough 2.Qi Deficiency-cough	9-15
1.Clear Heat 2.Nourish Body Fluids 3.Reduce swelling 4.Remove Pus	1.diabetes 2.Febrile Disease 3.skin lesion	"
1.Clear LU 2.Relieve chest discomfort	1.Phlegm obst.-chest fullness & distention 2.suppurative mastitis	12-30
1.Moisten Dryness 2.Lubricate Intestines	1.Body Fluid Deficiency -dry stools	9-15
1.Clear Heat, Resolve Phlegm	1.siezure, stroke delerium, mania	30-60

Hb Laminariae	Kun Bu 昆布	salty cold	LIV, ST KID	
Sargassum	Hai Zao 海藻	bitter salty cold	LU, SP KID, LIV	contra. with Rx Glycyrrhizae
Lapis Chloriti	Meng Shi 礞石	sweet salty neutral	LU, LIV	contra. pregnant
Rz Belamcandae	She Gan 射干	bitter cold toxic	"	contra. pregnant

1.Soften Hardenings 2.Diuretic	1.scrofula, T.B., lumps 2.edema, beriberi	"
1.Soften Hardenings 2.Promote Diuresis	1.goitre, scrofula TB of lymph nodes 2.chronic bronchitis 3.hypertension, edema	9-15
1.Subdue LIV 2.Anti-convulsive	1.epilepsy 2.convulsions	1.5-3
1.Clear Heat, Detoxify 2.Resolve phlegm, Soothe throat	1.tonsillitis, sore throat 2.cough, yellow mucous	6-9

CHAPTER 5

ANTI-TUSSIVE AND ANTI-ASTHMATIC HERBS

DEFINITION: Any herb that helps to arrest cough and stop asthma falls into this category.

GENERALIZATION: These herbs have Descending functions, hence deriving their actions to stop cough and asthma - both being the result of Rebellious Uprising Qi. Cough and asthma are very commmon conditions that have causes of both External and Internal origin, one must combine other appropriate methods and herbs and not overlook the causative and the complicating factors.

SYMPTOMATOLOGY: Cough and asthma are more like symptoms than conditions. Depending on the cause, one may see varied symptomatology. Commonly, cough and asthma may be caused by External Wind Cold or Wind Heat in which case they will be accompanied by fever and chills, body ache and either yellow or white phlegm, sometimes with facial edema.

If cough and asthma are caused by Qi Deficiency, one may see shortness of breath, fatique and chronic recurrence of the condition.

Other causes would be seen in Excess Cold or Heat, Cold Phlegm or Heat Phlegm Internally invading and obstructing the Lungs, consequently resulting in cough and asthma, chest discomfort and fullness, low appetite, white or yellow mucous, and etc.

CONTRAINDICATIONS: During the beginning stage of measles when cough is present, do not try to stop the cough by Descending or Astringing the Lung Qi, because this will enclose the pathogens within. Instead, one should Ventilate and Disperse the Lung Qi to expel the pathogenic factor.

PHARMOCOLOGICAL ACTIONS: Most herbs have been found clinically to be anti-tussive, antiasthmatic and expectorant in action. Some, in addition, have diuretic, antibiotic and laxative effects.

pharmaceutical name	pin-yin	taste & energy	meridians	comments
CATEGORY: ANTI-TUSSIVE & ANTI-ASTHMATIC HERBS				
Fl Farfarae	Kuan Dong Hua 款冬花	pungent warm	LU	
Fr Perilla Acutae	Zi Su Zi 紫蘇子	"	"	
Rx Stemonae	Bai Bu 百部	sweet bitter neutral	"	
Rx Asteris	Zi Wan 紫菀	bitter sweet sl.warm	"	
Cx Mori Radicis	Sang Bai Pi 桑白皮	sweet cold	"	
Fr Aristolochia	Ma Dou Ling 馬兜鈴	bitter sl.pung cold	LU, LI	
Sm Armeniacae	Xing Ren 杏仁	bitter sl.warm sl.tox.	"	
Fm Eriobotryae	Pi Pa Ye 枇杷葉	bitter neutral	LU, ST	

MAJOR ACTIONS: STOP COUGH, STOP ASTHMA		
secondary actions	symptoms/conditions	dose (g)
1.Descend LU Qi 2.Moisten LU	1.dry cough and many other coughs	3-9
1.Resolve Phlegm 2.Lubricate Intestines	1.Phlegm cough 2.constipation	"
1.Moisten LU 2.Anti-helmenthic	1.dry cough 2.tape worms-enema 3.pruritis, lice	"
1.Resolve Phlegm	1.Phlegm cough & other coughs	"
1.Clear LU Heat 2.Diuretic	1.LU Heat cough 2.edema, diff. urination 3.high blood presure	9-18
1.Clear LU, Resolve Phlegm 2.Lower blood pressure	1.LU Heat/LU def. cough 2.hemmorhoids 3.high blood presure	3-9
1.Descend LU Qi 2.Lubricate Intestines	1.any cough 2.constipation	"
1.Resolve Phlegm 2.Harmonize ST 3.Descend Rebellious ST Qi	1.Heat Phlegm cough 2.ST Heat-vomiting	9-15

CHAPTER 6

AROMATIC DAMPNESS RESOLVING HERBS

"The Earth Element has an affinity for warmth and fragrance."
                                                    - Ancient Classic

DEFINITION: Any herb that displays aromatic properties and has the action to dissolve and dry up Dampness falls into this category.

GENERALIZATION: Herbs in this category contain aromatic properties, that is, fragrant to the smell and have the ability to dry up pathogenic Damp factors that often than not, leads to Spleen dysfunction. They are mostly <u>pungent</u>, <u>warming</u>, and <u>drying</u> in nature and all enter the <u>Spleen</u>.
    Dampness in the body often affects the Spleen organ causing disturbance in the Spleen's function of regulating water matabolism. The Dampness can further weaken the Spleen, obstruct the Qi flow, and it can also join with other pathogenic factors such as Cold, Heat and Summer Heat. Therefore, it is crucial to strengthen the Spleen, regulate Qi flow, warm up the Interior, or clear the Heat at the same time when appropriate.

SYMPTOMATOLOGY: When Dampness hampers the Spleen's Transformation and Transportation function, it disturbs the gastrointestinal tract as follows: low appetite, fatigue, diarrhea, nausea, vomiting, epigastric and abdominal distension, "sickening" sweet taste in the mouth, white and greasy coating on the tongue and a slippery pulse.

CAUTIONS AND CONTRAINDICATIONS: Because herbs in this category are pungent, warm and dry, they tend to exhaust the Qi and drain the Yin and should be used with caution when the patient exhibits Deficiency in Yin, blood and Qi.
    In addition, since they all contain large amounts of volatile oils, when boiling the herb tea they are usually added later and then boiled for only a short time so that the desired effects are preserved.

PHARMACOLOGICAL ACTIONS: These herbs have been found, in laboratory and clinical research, to increase secretion of gastric juice, relieve the spasms of smooth muscles of the intestines, and antibiotic in action.

CATEGORY:	AROMATIC-DAMP RESOLVING HERBS			
pharmaceutical name	pin-yin	taste & energy	meridians	comments
Fr seu Sm Amomi	Sha Ren 砂仁	pungent warm	SP, ST KID	
Fr Amomi Cardamomi	Bai Dou Kou 白豆蔻	"	SP, ST	best if powered
Fr Amomi Tsaoko	Cao Guo 草果	"	"	
Sm Alpiniae Katsumadai	Cao Dou Kou 草豆蔻	"	"	
Rz Atractylodis	Cang Zhu 蒼朮	bitter pungent warm	"	good vit.A content use for Vit.A def. night-blindness
Cx Magnoliae Officinalis	Hou Po 厚朴	"	SP, ST LU, LI	
Hb Agastaches (Pogostemi)	Huo Xiang 藿香	pungent	SP, ST sl.warm LU	

MAJOR ACTIONS: WARM MIDDLE JIAO, RESOLVE DAMP		
secondary actions	symptoms/conditions	dose (g)
1. Invigorate Qi Flow 2. Stop diarrhea 3. Stabilize fetus	1. Qi Stagn. in Mid-Jiao 2. SP Def. diarrhea 3. fetal hypermotility	2-6
1. Invigorate Qi Flow 2. Stop vomiting	1. Damp Obstr. Qi Flow 2. vomiting, 3. ulcers	3-10 2-5powder
1. Dispel Phlegm 2. Relieve malaria	1. Phlegm Damp obstr MJ 2. malaria	3-6
1. Strengthen SP Yang 2. Stop vomiting	1. abd. fullness, low apetite 2. gastralgia, vomiting	2-6
1. Strengthen SP 2. Dispel Wind Damp 3. Diaphoretic	1. SP Deficiency 2. Wind Damp Bi 3. Wind Cold	3-10
1. Invigorate Qi Flow 2. Descend Rebellious Qi, Stop asthma	1. Qi Stagn. of MJ 2. asthma	3-9
1. Harmonize Middle Jiao 2. Stop vomiting 3. Diaphoretic	1. Damp retention 2. vomiting 3. Wind Cold + Int.Damp	3-10

CHAPTER 7

DIGESTIVE HERBS

DEFINITION: Any herb that aids in digestion, and relieves symtoms of indigestion is considered a Digestive herb.

GENERALIZATION: These herbs are all <u>sweet</u> in taste and enter the organs responsible for the digestive process of food, mainly the <u>Spleen</u> and the <u>Stomach</u>.
    More often than not, indigestion results from over eating, which over burdens the system and leads to food retention in the gastrointestinal tract. Secondary cause of indigestion stems from various pathogenic factors such as Cold and Damp, and also from a pre-existing weakness of Spleen and Stomach.
    To effectively resolve the problem, one must combine other appropriate herbs to a prescription such as Interior Warming herbs to dispel the Cold factor, Aromatic Damp Resolving herbs to dry up the Damp factor, Qi Regulating herbs to remove Qi Stagnation, Purgative herbs to relieve constipation and intestinal obstruction, and Spleen and Stomach Tonics for Deficiency.

SYMPTOMATOLOGY: Epigastric and abdominal fullness and distention, lack of appetite, belching, acid regurgitation, nausea, vomit, and irregular bowel movement such as constipation or diarrhea.

PHARMACOLOGICAL ACTIONS: These herbs have been found to increase the secretion of gastric juice and enhance the intestinal peristasis and evacuation.

CATEGORY: DIGESTIVE HERBS

pharmaceutical name	pin-yin	taste & energy	meridians	comments
Massa Fermenta	Shen Qu 神袖	sweet pungent	SP, ST	ingred.-fermented atractylodis alba, armeniaca, artemesia chinghao, phaesioli, red pepper, xanthium
Fr Oryzae	Gu Ya 谷芽	sweet neutral	"	
Fr Hordei	Mai Ya 麥芽	"	"	contra for nursing mother
Endothelium Corneum Gigeriae Galli	Ji Nei Jin 雞內金	"	SP, ST	better as powder
Sm Raphani	Lai Fu Zi 萊菔子	pungent sweet neutral	LU, SP ST	
Fr Cratagi	Shan Zha 山楂	sour sweet sl.warm	SP, ST LIV	

MAJOR ACTIONS: PROMOTE DIGESTION, RELIEVE STAGNANT FOOD		
secondary actions	symptoms/conditions	dose (g)
1.Strengthen ST	1.SP/ST Deficiency- diarrhea	10-15
1.Strengthen ST	1.Esp. good for "RICE" food retention	10-15
1.Strengthen ST 2.Help stop lactation	1."starchy" food reten. 2.undesired lactation	10-15 or (30-120)
1.Strengthen ST 2.Anti-ephidrotic 3.Dissolve stones	1.SP/ST Def-food reten. 2.enuresis, sem.emission 3.gall or UB stones	3-9
1.Relieve Distention 2.Resolve Phlegm 3.Descend Rebellious Qi	1.epig & abd distention 2.Phlegm Damp cough	6-12
1.Stregthen ST 2.Invigorate Blood 3.Remove Stagnation	1.esp. for "meat" Stagn 2.post-partum Blood Stagnation 3.hernia	10-15 or (30-120)

CHAPTER 8

QI REGULATING/CARMINATIVE HERBS

DEFINITION: Any herb that acts to disperse Qi Stagnation and facilitate Qi flow falls under this category.

GENERALIZATION: Most of these herbs are <u>pungent</u> and <u>warm</u> in nature. They all have, to different degrees, the ability to facilitate Qi flow, Soothe Liver, remove any Qi Stagnation, reverse Rebellious Qi activities (such as in cough, asthma and hiccups), and ensures Spleen functions. Some are stronger at Dispersing Stagnations, while others have actions of Resolving Phlegm and strengthening Spleen and Stomach.

Since the Liver organ is responsible in maintaining the patency, or the continuity of Qi flow in our body, most obstructions in Qi flow can be attributed to the malfunctioning of the Liver. In those cases, herbs to Soften and Guide the Liver are also to be used.

Realizing that a condition may be complicated by other pathogenic factors, one must be adaptive and use other herbs flexibly to attain the best results.

SYMPTOMATOLOGY: Qi Stagnation can occur in any area of the body, therefore, the corresponding symptomatology my vary. However, obvious symptoms are pain and distention. Most commonly, one may experience epigastric and abdominal fullness, distention and pain, nausea, vomiting, belching, constipation or inability to evacuate completely as a result of Qi Stagnation of Spleen and Stomach.

When the Liver Qi is obstructed, symptoms such as pain and distention in the hypochondriac area, epigastric bloating, acid regurgitation, depression, uncontrollable emotional out burst, irregular menstruation, breast distention and sensation of something like a plum pit lodged in the throat are experienced.

One may also encounter chest tightness, pressure and pain, cough, asthma and shortness of breath due to Lung Qi Stagnation.

CONTRAINDICATIONS: Noting that these herbs are pungent and warm, and may have a draining effect on Qi and Yin, one must use them with caution in cases of Qi and Yin Deficiency, or simultaneously with Yin or Qi tonics.

PHARMACOLOGICAL ACTIONS: Some herbs in this category have been found to stimulate the gastrointestinal tract, increase cardiac output, antiasthmatic and anti-inflammatory when administered in small doses.

	CATEGORY: CARMINATIVE HERBS			
pharmaceutical name	pin-yin	taste & energy	meridians	comments
Pericarpium Citri Reticulatae	Chen Pi 陳皮	pungent bitter warm	SP, LU	
Pericarpium Citri Reticulatae Viride	Qing Pi 青皮	"	LIV, GB ST	
Bulbus Allium	Xie Bai 薤白	"	LU, HT ST, LI	
Rx Saussureae	Mu Xiang 木香	"	SP, ST LI, GB	often used with tonics
Fr Citri Sarcodactylis	Fu Shou 佛手	"	LIV, SP LU	
Lignum Aquilaria	Chen Xiang 沉香	"	SP, ST KID	use as powder
Rx Linderae	Wu Yao 烏藥	pungent warm	ST, KID UB	
Lignum Santali Albi	Tan Xiang 檀香	"	SP, ST LU, HT	
Sm Litchi	Li Zhi He 荔枝核	"	LIV, ST	
Pericarpium Arecae	Da Fu Pi 大腹皮	pungent sl.warm	SP, ST SI, LI	

MAJOR ACTIONS: INVIGORATE QI FLOW, REMOVE STAGNATION		
secondary actions	symptoms/conditions	dose (g)
1.Tonify SP 2.Dry Damp & Phlegm 3.Descend Rebellious Qi	1.SP Def. with Damp 2.Phlegm-Damp in chest 3.vomiting	3-9
1.Smooth LIV Qi 2.Remove Qi Stagnation	1.LIV Qi Stagnation 2.Blood Stagnation	3-9
1.Stop pain 2.Invigorate Yang Qi	1.Cold Stagnation in abdomen	9-15
1.Stop pain	1.GB colics	3-9
1.Stop pain 2.Harmonize ST 3.Resolve Phlegm	1.LIV Qi Stagnation 2.Phlegm-Damp in chest	3-9
1.Stop pain 2.Disperse Cold 3.Descend Rebellious Qi, Relieve asthma	1.vomiting 2.Cold ST	1-3
1.Disperse Cold 2.Stop pain	1.Lower Jiao Cold frequent urination 2.hernia	3-12
1.Stop pain 2.Disperse Cold 3.Improve appetite	1.Blood Stagnation pain 2.ST Cold	1-3
1.Disperse Cold 2.Stop pain 3.Disperse Hardenings	1.hernia 2.Blood Stagnation in abdomen	.2-.4
1.Remove food Stagnation 2.Diuretic	1.food retention 2.edema	3-9

Fr Ponciri (Fr. Aurantii Immaturis)	Zhi Shi 枳實	bitter pungent sl.sour sl.warm	SP, ST	
Fr Aurantii	Zhi Ke 枳殼	"	SP, ST	milder function than Fr Ponceri
Rz Cyperi	Xiang Fu 香附	pungent sl.bit. neutral	LIV, ST	
Calyx Kaki	Shi Di 柿蒂	bitter neutral	ST	
Fr Meliae Toosendan	Chuan Lian Zi 川楝子	bitter cold toxic	LIV, SI UB	overdose can cause paralysis

1. Resolve Phlegm 2. Disperse Hardenings	1. Phlegm-Damp in Middle Jiao 2. constipation 3. organ prolapse	3-9 or 12 30 for prolapse
1. Relieve distention	1. epigastric & abdominal distention	3-9
1. Smooth LIV Qi 2. Regulate menses, Stop pain	1. LIV Qi Stagnation 2. irregular menses, dysmenorrhea	6-12
1. Descend Rebellious Qi	1. ST Cold-belching	3-9
1. Anti-helmenthic 2. Stop pain	1. worms 2. Cold Stagnation-pain	10-15

CHAPTER 9

DOWNWARD DISCHARGING HERBS

DEFINITION: Any herb that aids in moving the stools, relieves constipation, acts on the Lower Jiao(Heater) of the body and excretes water retention in the chest or abdominal cavities falls into this category.

GENERALIZATION: There are 3 subcategories of Downward Discharging herbs. They are: 1) Purgative herbs 2) Lubricant herbs and 3) Cathartic Diuretic herbs. They are mainly used in Excess conditions, although the Lubricant herbs are often used in constipation due to Deficient conditions.

Because of the potent actions, Downward Discharging herbs, mainly the Purgatives and Cathartic Diuretic herbs, are avoided in cases of pregnancy, excess menstruation and old and weak patients. In addition, these herbs tend to purge and damage the Stomach Qi, thus, one must closely regulate the duration and the amount of usage to avoid causing side effects.

In multi-syndrome conditions such as External condition with Internal condition existing simultaneously, one must relieve the External condition first, or if necessary, one may chose to treat the External and Internal ailment at the same time, so as not to drive pathogens deeper into the body. This same priciple can be applied to conditions of Excess (pathogen) and Deficiency (body) at the same time. By combining with Tonic herbs, one can prevent further injuring and draining of the body's Original Qi.

SECTION ONE

PURGATIVE HERBS

"The six Fu organs are hollow in structure, thus they must remain hollow and clear of any obstruction for proper functioning."
                                                    - Ancient Classic

"To extinguish the blazing fire, simply remove the logs from underneath."
                                                    - Ancient Classic

DEFINITION: Any herb that has the actions of loosen the stools, relieve constipation, disperse stagnation and purge Excess Heat from the body is considered a Pugative herb.

GENERALIZATION: Herbs in this category are <u>bitter</u> and <u>cold</u> and enter the <u>Large Intestine Channels</u>, thus they have <u>Descending</u> and <u>Cooling</u> properties. Frequently, they are combined with Qi Regulating herbs, and Heat Clearing herbs to enhance the purging and laxative effect. Sometimes, they are employed for their purging actions in cases of Excess Cold Stagnation in the Lower Jiao(Heater) together with Interior Warming herbs. These herbs are more recently used in cases of acute abdomen.

SYMPTOMATOLOGY: The application of purgative herbs are immense. Not only are they useful in obstruction of the bowels, as in constipation, but also in Excess Heat conditions, particularly when the Fire Blazes Upwardly, not necessarily exhibiting constipation at all. These herbs are also beneficial in dysentery of the Excess Heat type and are frequently used together with Antihelminthic herbs for maximal effects.

Excess Heat in the Intestines will dry up the fluids and harden the stools causing constipation, abdominal fullness, bloating and pain, foul breath, red tongue with thick and yellow coat.

Fire in the upper part of the body will display some of the following symptoms: high fever, delirium, hysteria, mania, flushed face, headache, red eyes, sore throat, swollen bleeding gums, and hemorrhaging in the upper body such as epistaxis, hemoptysis, and hematemesis. (Here, utilizing the principle stated above - to extinguish the Blazing Fire, one simply remove the logs from underneath.)

When Heat and Damp factors combine to accumulate in the Intestines, one will most likely develop acute dysentery with tenesmus, foul smelling stools with burning sensation in the anus, yellow greasy tongue coating with rapid and slippery pulse.

CONTRAINDICATIONS: Due to their drastic actions, Purgative herbs are contra-indicated in pregnancy, old and Deficient patients.

PHARMACOLOGICAL ACTIONS: These herbs have been found to have antibiotic, laxative and antitoxin effects.

SECTION TWO

LUBRICANT HERBS

DEFINITION: Any herb that helps to lubricate the body and relieve constipation without involving purging actions are considered to be a Lubricant herb.

GENERALIZATION: Lubricant herbs are <u>sweet</u> in nature because they Tonify somewhat, by lubricating and regenerating Body Fluids, and of course, they all enter the <u>Large Intestines</u> channel.

SYMPTOMATOLOGY: These herbs are commonly applied in constipation and dry stools in elderly patients that are Deficient in Body Fluids, postpartum anemia, and persons recovering from a Febrile disease. Most often, Yin Tonics, Blood Tonics, and Heat Clearing herbs are implemented to effectively treat the conditions.

PHARMACOLOGICAL ACTIONS: Herbs in this category are similar to other herb seeds in that they contain a high proportion of fatty acids that can stimulate the intestinal mucosa and increase peristalsis.

SECTION THREE

CATHARTIC DIURETIC HERBS

DEFINITION: Any herb that purges excessive water accumulation from the body, sometimes violently, through urination and defecation is considered to be a Cathartic Diuretic.

GENERALIZATION: These herbs are potent and toxic and will elicit the body's response to excrete water, sometimes in a violent manner and can cause diarrhea, thus, it is crucial to understand its working mechanism so as not to cause any side effects. They are generally useful in cases of fluid retention in the abdomen (as in ascites), and chest (as in pulmonary edema and pleurisy). However, it is important to carefully monitor the strength of both the patient and the pathogen to help determine the addition of Tonic herbs at appropriate times.

SYMPTOMATOLOGY: Please see below for the symptomatology.

TABLE 7 - WATER RETENTION OF THE CHEST AND ABDOMEN

CONDITION	SIGNS AND SYMPTOMS
WATER ACCUMULATION IN THE CHEST	cough, asthma, dyspnea, chest fullness and distention, coughing up copious white sputum, chest and hypochondriac pain, sometimes even seizures may occur
WATER ACCUMULATION IN THE ABDOMEN	abdominal swelling, difficult urination edema of lower limbs, distention and bloating, sometimes pain in the abdomen

CONTRAINDICATIONS: Due to their drastic actions and the fact that most of the herbs in this category are toxic, Cathartic Diuretics are contraindicated in pregnant woman, old and weak patients, Yin and Qi Deficiency and prolonged intake.

PHARMACOLOGICAL ACTIONS: These herbs promote purgation and diuresis in lab animals. Some also have cardiotonic effects.

CATEGORY: PURGATIVE HERBS				
pharmaceutical name	pin-yin	taste & energy	meridians	comments
Rz Rhei	Da Huang 大黃	bitter cold	SP, ST LI, LIV PER	contra preg,menstr, lactating. avoid overcooking
Hb Aloes	Lu Hui 蘆薈	"	LIV, LI ST	contra pregnant
Fm Sennae	Fan Xie Ye 番瀉葉	sweet bitter cold	LI	contra pregnant overdose causes nausea & vomiting
Mirabilitum Depuratum (Sodium Sulfate)	Mang Xiao 芒硝	bitter salty cold	ST, LI	contra pregnant no need to cook extremely cold
Sm Ricini	Bi Ma Zi 蓖麻子	sweet pungent neutral toxic	"	contra pregnant

CATEGORY: LUBRICANT HERBS				
pharmaceutical name	pin-yin	taste & energy	meridians	comments
Sm Cannabis	Huo Ma Ren 火麻仁	sweet neutral	SP, ST LI	overdose causes dizziness & vertigo
Sm Pruni	Yu Li Ren 郁李仁	sweet bitter neutral	LI, SI	contra pregnant

MAJOR ACTIONS: PURGE HEAT, REMOVE CONSTIPATION

secondary actions	symptoms/conditions	dose (g)
1.Cool Blood 2.Invigorate Blood, Remove Stagn. 3.Benefit GB	1.Blood Heat-bleeding 2.Blood Stagnation 3.Damp Heat jaundice	3-12
1.Anti-helmenthic	1.worms (intestinal) 2.Excess LIV Fire	1-2
1.Drain Summer Heat	1.Excess Heat constip.	3-6
1.Soften Hardenings	1.dry stool 2.acute appendicitis 3.skin disease (ext)	10-15
1.Resolve abscess	1.food retention, constipation, abscess boils, carbuncles, skin lesions	1.5-3

MAJOR ACTIONS: LUBRICATE INTESTINES, RELIEVE CONSTIPATION

secondary actions	symptoms/conditions	dose (g)
1.Lubricate Intestines, Relieve constipation 2.Nourish Body Fluids	1.Body Fluid Def. 2.Yin Def.	9-30
1.Lubricate Intestines, Relieve constipation 2.Diuretic	1.edema 2.dysuria	3-12

CATEGORY:	CATHARDIC	DIURETIC	HERBS	
pharmaceutical name	pin-yin	taste & energy	meridians	comments
Sm Crotonis	Ba Dou 巴豆	pungent hot toxic	LIV, LI KID	contra pregnant contra with Sm Pharbitides very toxic
Sm Euphorbiae Lathyridis	Xu Sui Zi 續隨子	pungent warm toxic	"	contra pregnant
Hb Euphorbiae Pekinensis	Da Ji 大戟	bitter cold toxic	LU, LI KID	contra pregnant contra with Rx Glycyrrhiza
Rx Euphorbiae Kansui	Gan Sui 甘遂	"	"	contra pregnant contra with Rx Glycyrrhizae
Sm Pharbitides	Qian Niu Zi 牽牛子	bitter pungent cold toxic	LU, KID LI, SI	contra. pregnant caution SP/ST Def.
Rx Phytolaccae	Shang Lu 商陸	bitter pungent neutral toxic	"	contra pregnant

MAJOR ACTIONS: PURGE WATER ACCUMULATION

secondary actions	symptoms/conditions	dose (g)
1. Remove Water accumulation Promote urination 2. Resolve Phlegm 3. Benefit throat 4. Pus eruptions	1. Lower Jiao Cold Stagnation 2. Phlegm Stagnation 3. skin disease	.1-.3
1. Remove Water accumulation 2. Invigorate Blood, Remove Stagnation	1. tumors	1.5-3
1. Remove Water accumulation 2. Reduce swelling 3. Disperse Stagnation	1. skin disease (ext)	1.5-3
1. Remove Water accumulation 2. Reduce swelling, Disperse Hardenings	1. abd. water retention difficult urination & B.M. 2. pulm. edema, plurisy	.5-1
1. Remove water accumulation 2. Anti-helminthic 3. Relieve constipation	1. edema, oliguria 2. ascariasis 3. constipation	4-9
1. Remove Water accumulation 2. Resolve Phlegm, Stop cough 3. Detoxify, Reduce swelling	1. Cold Phlegm-cough 2. skin disease (ext)	4-9

CHAPTER 10

ANTIHELMINTHIC HERBS

DEFINITION: Any herb that has the ability to kill or inhibit worms, parasites and fungi is called an Antihelminthic herb.

GENERALIZATION: Some of these herbs are <u>toxic</u> and are used mainly for intestinal worms and parasites, although they are also useful in other affected areas of the body. Normally, they are taken on an empty stomach to ensure maximal results in disabling the intestinal worms or parasites and also taken with Purgatives to properly excrete the culprits out of the body.

Generally, depending on the accompanied symptoms, one would also combine herbs from such categories as Digestives, Spleen and Stomach Tonics, and Qi Regulators in appropriate conditions.

SYMPTOMATOLOGY: Intestinal worms are frequently introduced by unsanitary and raw foods. One may display abdominal pain and bloating, nausea, vomiting, enormous or no appetite, an affinity to eat strange substances, itching in the anus, nose and ears, sallow facial complexion, emaciation or edema, and spots in the sclera of the eyes.

Parasites and worms of other sorts can take up residence in other parts of the body such as the vagina, skin and the like. In these instance, one may chose to apply the herbs both externally and internally.

Example of some of the conditions include round worms, pin worms, tape worms, hook worms, trichomonas, etc.

CAUTIONS AND CONTRAINDICATIONS: Because some herbs are toxic, one should use them with caution in pregnant women, old and weak patients.

PHARMACOLOGICAL ACTIONS: These herbs are antiparasitic, antifungal, antiviral and antibacterial in action.

	CATEGORY:	ANTIHELMINTHIC HERBS		
pharmaceutical name	pin-yin	taste & energy	meridians	comments
Sm Arecae	Bing Lang 檳榔	pungent bitter warm	ST,LI	
Fr Quisqualis	Shi Jun Zi 使君子	sweet warm	SP, ST	can be taken raw overdose causes nausea & vomiting
Sm Hydnocarpi	Da Feng Zi 大風子	pungent hot toxic	ST, SP LIV	
Lythargyrum	Mi Tuo Shen 蜜陀僧	pungent salty neutral toxic	SP, ST	ext. use only
Melanteritum	Lu Fan 綠矾	sour cold	"	
Sm Torreyae	Fei Zi 榧子	sweet astrng neutral	ST, LI	
Calomelas	Qing Fen 輕粉	pungent cold toxic	LIV, KID UB	contra pregnant
Nidus Vespae	Feng Fang 蜂房	sweet neutral toxic	LU, LIV ST	do not use on open wounds

80

MAJOR ACTIONS: KILL WORMS & PARASITES

secondary actions	symptoms/conditions	dose (g)
1.Anti-helminthic 2.Carminative 3.Diuretic	1.many types of worms 2.Qi Stagnation 3.beriberi	6-15
1.Anti-helminthic	1.round worms, tape worms	6-15
1.Anti-helminthic 2.Dispel Wind	1.ext.-fungal infection parasites 2.int.-leprosy	.3-.5
1.Anti-helminthic 2.Dry Damp 3.Aid wound healing	1.eczema,tinea,genital itching 2.strong underarm odor	3-30
1.Anti-helminthic 2.Dry Damp 3.Nourish Blood (in small dose)	1.worms, eczema 2.obesity 3.anemia	.1-.3
1.Anti-helminthic 2.Stop diarrhea	1.intestinal worms 2.diarrhea, dysentery	15-30
1.Detoxify (Ext.) 2.Promote Diuresis	1.scabies,tinea,neuro-dermatitis,syphilitic chancres 2.edema,scanty urination, constipation	.1-.2
1.Dispel Internal Wind 2.Detoxify	1.convulsions 2.urticaria, tumor, chronic cough 3.suppurative skin lesion, pain & swelling of gums	3-5

CHAPTER 11

AROMATIC STIMULANT HERBS

DEFINITION: Any herb that Opens the Orifices and Awakens consciousness with its pungent, aromatic properties is called an Aromatic Stimulant herbs.

GENERALIZATION: These herbs can be compared to the smelling salts of the conventional medicine in that they are also _aromatic_ in nature. The _pungent_ taste disperses any Stagnation and Opens the Orifice so that one's Spirit may function again.

There are mainly two types of sudden coma. One is called the "closed" type in which the symptoms are characterized by tightness, contraction and stagnation. The other is typically like shock in that substance and energy are drained from the body. This is called the "open" type of coma.

Since the herbs in this category act to "open" and disperse any obstructions of the orifice, they are used in the "closed" type and NOT the "open" type of unconsciousness.

Please see below for the differentiation.

SYMPTOMATOLOGY: Table 8 lists the two types of unconscious conditions.

TABLE 8 - DIFFERENTIATION OF UNCONSCIOUSNESS

TYPE	CONDITION	SIGNS AND SYMPTOMS	TREATMENT
CLOSED	Heat	high fever, red face unconsciousness, eyes closed, teeth clenched tight fist, P-rapid and full, T-yellow coat	Opens Orifice Cools Fire
	Cold	cyanosis, cold body, unconsciousness, eyes closed, teeth clenched tight fist, P-slow and deep, T-White coat	Opens Orifice Warm Up Cold
OPEN	Collapse of Yang	unconsciousness, cold body, profuse sweat P-feeble and faint	Restore Yang Reinforce Qi

CAUTIONS AND CONTRAINDICATIONS: These herbs are contraindicated in the OPEN TYPE of unconsciousness. And because of the dispersing quality that is so crucial in these herbs, they are not boiled as a tea but instead are taken in pill or powder form.

PHARMACOLOGICAL ACTIONS: These herbs are known to stimulate the central nervous system to revive from unconsciousness, elevate blood pressure, and increase digestive secretion. Some of the herbs also have sedative effects.

CATEGORY: AROMATIC STIMULANT HERBS				
pharmaceutical name	pin-yin	taste & energy	meridians	comments
Rz Acori Graminei	Chang Pu 菖蒲	pungent warm	HT, ST	
Moschus	She Xiang 麝香	"	HT, SP	contra pregnant
Styrax Liquidius	Su He Xiang 蘇合香	"	"	use as powder
Benzoinum	An Xi Xiang 安息香	pungent bitter neutral	"	use as powder
Borneolum	Bing Pian 冰片	pungent bitter cool	HT, LU	contra pregnant
Calculus Bovis	Niu Huang 牛黄	bitter sweet cool	LIV, HT	contra pregnant

MAJOR ACTIONS: CLEAR ORIFICES, RESTORE CONCIOUSNESS

secondary actions	symptoms/conditions	dose (g)
1.Aromatic, Dry Damp 2.Calm Spirit	1.Middle Jiao Damp 2.manic, hysteria, poor memory	3-10 or 10-15- fresh
1.Invigorate Blood 2.Disperse Hardenings 3.Induce abortion 4.Detoxify	1.traumas, tumors amenorrhea 2.dead fetus 3.skin lesions	0.1-0.15
1.Activate Blood flow	1.angina	0.3-1

1.Resolve Phlegm
2.Invigorate Qi & Blood
	1.Phlegm obstructing
	  Orifices
	2.Qi & Blood Stagnation-
	  epig. & abd. pain
		0.3-1

1.Dispel Heat, Stop pain	1.high fever causing
	  unconciousness &
	  convulsions
	2.pharyngitis,tonsil-
	  itis,laryngitis,
	  stomatitis
		.03-.1

1.Calm LIV Wind
2.Relieve convulsions
3.Resolve Phlegm
4.Clear Orifices
5.Clear Heat, Detoxify
	1.LIV Wind due to
	  excess Heat
	2.throat inflammation
	  skin lesions
		0.15-3

CHAPTER 12

INTERIOR WARMING HERBS

DEFINITION: Any herb that has the ability to warm up the Interior and dispel Cold factors falls into this category.

GENERALIZATION: These herbs are <u>pungent</u> and <u>warm</u> in nature and most of them enter the <u>Spleen</u> and <u>Kidney</u> channels. There are two main avenues where the pathogenic Cold can affect the body. One is the invasion of pathogenic Cold from the Exterior of the body which commonly settles in the Middle Jiao (Heater) and disturbs the digestive processes; another arises from a Deficiency of Yang, mainly that of the Kidneys which fail to keep the body warm and consequently results in a Cold condition. Interior Warming herbs act to take care of both causes by warming the Middle Jiao and dispelling the Cold, strengthening the Fire and benefiting the Yang.

However, one must always remember to distinguish other factors that may be complicating the condition and combine proper herbs with the Interior Warming herbs to achieve the treatment goal.

SYMPTOMATOLOGY: Cold conditions in the Interior has two causes, one arises from pathogenic Cold Invasion, the other due to Insufficiency of body's Yang.

TABLE 9 — EXCESS AND DEFICIENT COLD

CONDITION	SIGNS AND SYMPTOMS	MAY COMBINE WITH
COLD INVASION	pale face, nausea, diarrhea, epigastric and abdominal pain and coldness, likes heat, no appetite, achy limbs vomiting, P-tense	Qi Regulating herbs Damp Resolving herb Spleen and Stomach Tonic herbs
YANG DEFICIENCY	Coldness, edema, cold sweat, fatigue, rapid breathing, frequent urination, impotence P-faint and frail	Qi Tonic herbs Yang Tonic herbs

CAUTIONS AND CONTRAINDICATIONS: Herbs in this category are for warming purpose, are hot in nature and easily damage the Yin and Body Fluids. Therefore, use them with caution for Yin, Blood, and Body Fluid Deficient patients.

PHARMACOLOGICAL ACTIONS: These herbs have been found to have cardiotonic, vasodilatory and analgesic effects. Some of the herbs can increase blood pressure while others have effect of lowering the blood pressure.

CATEGORY: INTERIOR WARMING HERBS

pharmaceutical name	pin-yin	taste & energy	meridians	comments
Fr Piperis Longi	Bi Ba 蓽撥	pungent hot	ST, LI	
Fr Piperis	Hu Qiao 胡椒	"	"	use as powder
Rz Alpiniae Officinalis	Gao Liang Jiang 高良姜	"	SP, ST	
Rz Zingiberis (dry)	Gan Jiang 干姜	"	SP, ST HT, LU	contra pregnant
Cx Cinnamomi	Rou Gui 肉桂	pungent sweet hot	KID, SP HT, LIV	contra pregnant don't overcook
Rx Aconiti Carm. Praeparata	Fu Zi 附子	pungent sweet hot toxic	HT, SP KID	contra pregnant
Fr Evodiae	Wu Zhu Yu 吳茱萸	pungent bitter hot toxic	LIV, KID SP, ST	overdose may cause visual disturbance
Fr Foeniculi	Xiao Hui Xiang 小茴香	pungent warm	"	
Fl Caryophylli	Ding Xiang 丁香	"	SP, ST	do not use with Rz Curcuma
Fr Zanthoxyli	Hua Jiao (Chuan Jiao) 花椒	pungent hot, sl. toxic	"	

MAJOR ACTIONS: WARM MIDDLE JIAO, DISPEL INTERNAL COLD		
secondary actions	symptoms/conditions	dose (g)
1.Stop vomiting	1.ST Cold	1-3
1.Antidote for food poisoning	1.Middle Jiao Cold	0.5-1
1.Stop pain 2.Stop vomiting	1.Middle Jiao Cold 2.vomiting	3-5
1.Restore Yang 2.Warm Lu, Resolve sputum	1.Yang Deficiency 2.Middle Jiao Cold 3.LU Cold cough	3-9
1.Tonify KID Yang 2.Stop pain	1.KID Yang Deficiency 2.Cold Stagn-abd. pain, dysmenorrhea	2-5
1.Retore Yang in emergency 2.Warm KID Yang 3.Relieve pain	1.shock 2.Collapse of Yang 3.Cold Damp Bi	3-9
1.Descend Rebellious Qi, Stop vomiting 2.Stop pain	1.vomiting 2.ST Cold	2-6
1.Regulate Qi, Harmonize ST 2.Stop pain	1.ST Cold 2.hernia	3-8
1.Descend Rebellious Qi 2.Warm KID Yang	1.ST Cold 2.KID Yang Deficiency	1-3
1.Stop pain 2.Anti-helminthic	1.Middle Jiao Cold 2.worms	2-5

CHAPTER 13

LIVER PACIFYING HERBS

DEFINITION: Any herb that has the capability of Pacifying Liver, Subduing Liver Fire and Calming Liver Wind falls into this category.

GENERALIZATION: This category of herbs is particular in that it works mainly on Liver disharmonies, thus they all enter the Liver Channel. Because the Liver has a tendency towards Heat conditions in pathology, whether it's Liver Fire Blazing, Liver Yang Rising or Liver Yin Deficient Fire, these herbs correspondingly are mostly Cold or Cooling. In addition, Liver in Five Element (or Five Phase) theory, being the Wood element receives its lubrication and nourishment from the Water element which corresponds to salty taste. We then observe that a good portion of Liver Pacifying herbs are salty.

Here, we separate this category of herbs into two, more specific subcategories that target at the distinctive features of Liver pathology. One is called the Liver Yang Sedative herbs and the other Liver Wind Calming herbs.

PHARMACOLOGICAL ACTIONS: These herbs sedate the central nervous system to promote anticonvulsive, sedative and antihypertensive effects. Some have also been found to have vasodilatory effect.

SECTION ONE

LIVER WIND CALMING HERBS

DEFINITION: Any herb that is capable of calming and arresting Liver Wind and relieve tremors, spasms and convulsions is considered a Liver Wind Calming herb.

GENERALIZATION: These herbs have actions of calming and stopping Liver Wind. The pathogenic Wind most often stems from a Heat source in the body, mainly that of Liver Yang Rising, it then travels in the channels and collaterals causing tremors and spasms and convulsions. When severe, the Wind will "shut the door" of the Heart Orifice and consequently result in coma, delirium or unconsciousness.

One will notice that many of the herbs in this category are insects such as scorpion, centipede, earth worm and silk worm. The reason being that these insects and worms are said to be capable of crawling in the channels and collaterals, absorbing and calming the Wind, thus relieving the spasms, tremors and convulsions. And when necessary, they will unobstruct the orifices to restore consciousness.

Liver Wind Calming herbs are often complemented with Liver Yang Sedative herbs to enhence the effects.

SYMPTOMATOLOGY: Wind is characterized in nature by sudden motion, constantly moving, and always changing and unpredictable. We also see Wind in the body manifesting signs and symptoms as tremors, spasms, convulsions, difficult speech, tetany, stiff neck, vertigo, ringing in the ears, twitching; and when severe, unconsciousness. Wind can be further complicated by joining with other pathogenic factors such as Phlegm. Some of the following conditions correspond to the pathology of Liver Wind: stroke, tetanus, seizures, and epilepsy.

CAUTIONS AND CONTRAINDICATIONS: Some of these herbs are toxic and should not be used during pregnancy.

SECTION TWO

LIVER YANG SEDATIVE HERBS

DEFINITION: Any herb that sedates and subdues the Uprising of Liver Yang falls into this category.

GENERALIZATION: These herbs not only function in sedating and subduing the Exuberance of Liver Yang, some of them also calm the Spirit and clear the Liver. Most of the herbs in this category are shells and bones that have heavy mineral content as to push down the rising Liver Yang. And because Heat often causes Internal Wind, these herbs are often supplemented with Liver Wind Calming herbs.

SYMPTOMATOLOGY: In Traditional Chinese Medicine, the Liver, among all other organs, is most prone to flare up with Heat conditions. This can be readily seen in people displaying fits of anger and uncontrollable emotions. The Yang of the Liver has a tendency to be Excess while the Yin has the tendency to be insufficient.

On the next page, table 10 lists the various Liver Heat conditions and their symptomatology.

TABLE 10 - LIVER HEAT SYNDROMES

CONDITION	SIGNS & SYMPTOMS	TX PRINCIPLE
LIVER FIRE BLAZING	feverish, severe headache red painful and swollen eyes vertigo, uncontrollable emotional out burst, anger severe ear ringing P-full, rapid and wiry T-red and dry, yellow coat	Purge LV fire Clear LIV Sedate LIV Yang
LIVER YANG RISING	intermittent feverish sensation in upper body, moderate headache, red painful eyes ringing in the ear, dizzy anger or depression, P-rapid and wiry T-red, yellow coat	Sedate LIV Yang Calm LIV Wind
LIVER YIN DEF. HEAT	low grade afternoon fever feverish palms, soles and chest, irritability, figid photophobia, night blindness blurry & dry eyes, dizziness ringing in the ear, P-thready and rapid, T-red, thin coat	Nourish Yin Sedate LIV Yang

CAUTIONS AND CONTRAINDICATIONS: Most herbs in this category are from minerals or bones and are more difficult to extract their content. Therefore, it is advisable to precook them one half to one hour before boiling the rest of the herbs in a prescription.

93

CATEGORY: LIVER WIND CALMING HERBS

pharmaceutical name	pin-yin	taste & energy	meridians	comments
Lumbricus	Di Long 地龍	salty cold	LIV, SP UB	use as powder
Cornu Antelopis	Ling Yang Jiao 羚羊角	"	LIV, HT	use as powder
Concha Haliotidis	Shi Jue Ming 石决明	"	LIV	
Scolopendra	Wu Gong 蜈蚣	salty toxic warm	"	contra pregnant large dose harmful
Rz Gastrodia	Tien Ma 天麻	sweet neutral	"	use as powder
Fr Tribuli	Bai Ji Li (Ci Ji Li) 白蒺藜	bitter pungent neutral	"	
Scorpio	Quan Xie 全蝎	salty pungent neutral toxic	"	contra Blood Def.
Bombyx Batryticatus	Jiang Can 僵蚕	salty pungent neutral	LIV, LU	use fresh for Wind Heat, fried for all other uses
Rm Uncarriae	Gou Teng 鈎藤	sweet sl.cold	LIV, P	don't overcook

MAJOR ACTIONS: CALM LIVER WIND, RELIEVE CONVULSION

secondary actions	symptoms/conditions	dose (g)
1.Clear Heat 2.Relieve asthma 3.Invigorate Collaterals 4.Ease urination	1.mental disorders 2.LU Heat asthma 3.Heat Bi 4.dysuria	5-15
1.Brighten eyes 2.Clear Heat, Detoxify	1.LIV Fire - red & painful eyes 2.Ying & Xue stage Heat	1-3
1.Subdue LIV Yang 2.Clear LIV 3.Brighten eyes	1.LIV Yang Rising 2.eye disorders	15-30
1.Detoxify 2.Disperse Hardenings 3.Invigorate Collaterals 4.Stop pain	1.infantile convulsion 2.skin lesions 3.Bi syndrome 4.chronic headache	1-3 or 0.6-1- powder
1.Subdue LIV Yang 2.Dispel Wind Damp	1.LIV Yang Rising 2.Bi syndrome	3-9
1.Subdue LIV Yang 2.Smooth LIV 3.Dispel Wind, Brighten eyes	1.LIV Yang Rising 2.LIV Qi Stagnation 3.red & painful eyes 4.itching	6-10
1.Detoxify, Resolve Hardenings 2.Invigorate Qi, Relieve pain	1.tics, convulsions, infantile convulsion 2.after stroke 3.abscess, scrofula 4.migraine, Bi pain	2-5
1.Dispel Wind 2.Resolve Phlegm 3.Stop pain 4.Disperse hardenings	1.Wind Heat 2.Phlegm Heat induced convulsion 3.scrofula, etc.	3-10
1.Clear Heat 2.Subdue LIV Yang	1.LIV Yang Rising 2.hypertension	10-15

CATEGORY:	LIVER YANG SEDATIVE HERBS			
pharmaceutical name	pin-yin	taste & energy	meridians	comments
Magnetitum	Ci Shi 磁石	salty cold	LIV, HT KID	contra SP, ST Def.
Margaritifera	Zhen Zhu 珍珠母	"	LIV, HT	
Os Draconis	Long Gu 龍骨	sweet sl.cold astring	"	
Hematitum	Dai Zhe Shi 代赭石	bitter cold	"	contra pregnant
Concha Ostrea	Mu Li 牡蠣	salty sl.cold	LIV, KID	

MAJOR ACTIONS: **SUBDUE LIVER YANG**		
secondary actions	symptoms/conditions	dose (g)
1.Tonify KID 2.Relieve asthma 3.Benefit hearing & vision	1.KID Def.-asthma 2.tinnitus, deafness, blurry vision	9-30
1.Clear LIV 2.Brighten eyes	1.red eyes, blurry vision	15-60
1.Calm Spirit 2.Astringent	1.insomnia, mania 2.nocturnal emission, spontaneous sweat	15-30
1.Descend Rebellious Qi 2.Hemostatic	1.belching, vomiting, asthma 2.Blood Heat-bleeding	10-30

1.Soften Hardenings
2.Astringent
	1.lymph node, liver or
	   spleen enlargement
	2.nocturnal emission,
	   spontaneous sweat
	3.peptic ulcer
		15-30

CHAPTER 14

SPIRIT TRANQUILIZING HERBS

DEFINITION: Any herb that calms the Spirit is referred to as a Spirit Tranquilizing herb.

GENERALIZATION: Herbs in this category strengthen the Heart and calms the Spirit. Most of them are <u>sweet</u> and all enter the <u>Heart</u> channel.

In Traditional theory, there are many causes of a disturbed Spirit. Some are due to weakness, others are caused by pathogenic factors such as Heat and Wind. Regarding the causes, one must not depend solely on spirit tranquilizing herbs, but rather one must add other appropriate herbs to a prescription to treat the cause. The causes and their corresponding treatments can be found in the Symptomatology section.

SYMPTOMATOLOGY: When the Spirit is disturbed, one will manifest instability in comprehension, emotions and the consciousness. It will also affect the physical heart causing such symptoms as palpitations. Other symptoms include insomnia, irritability, anxiety, fear, poor memory, hysteria, mania, and seizures.

The causes are numerous and the following table will give the corresponing treatment principle.

TABLE 11 — CAUSES OF SPIRIT DISTURBANCE

CAUSE	TREATMENT PRICIPLE
HEART QI DEFICIENCY	Tonify Heart Qi, Calm the Spirit
HEART BLOOD DEFICIENCY	Nourish Heart Blood, Calm the Spirit
HEART YIN DEF. HEAT	Nourish Heart Yin, Clear False Heat and Calm the Spirit
HEART FIRE BLAZING	Clear Heart Fire, Calm the Spirit
LIVER YANG RISING	Sedate Liver Yang, Calm the Spirit
PHLEGM MISTING THE HEART	Resolve Phlegm, Open the Orifice Calm the Spirit
WIND DISTURBING THE HEART	Pacify Liver, Calm the Wind

CAUTIONS AND CONTRAINDICATIONS: Some of the herbs have lubricating effect and are contraindicated in patients with diarrhea.

PHARMACOLOGICAL ACTIONS: Some of the herbs have sedative and antihypertensive effects.

CATEGORY: SPIRIT TRANQUILIZING HERBS				
pharmaceutical name	pin-yin	taste & energy	meridians	comments
Sm Biota	Bai Zi Ren 柏子仁	sweet neutral	HT, KID LI	
Fl et Cx Albizziae	He Huan Pi 合歡皮	"	HT, LIV	use both Fl & Cx for Qi Stagn. Cx only for trauma & lung abcess
Caulis Polygoni Multiflori	Ye Jiao Teng 夜交藤	"	"	
Sm Zizyphi Spinosa	Suan Zao Ren 酸棗仁	sweet sour neutral	"	
Cinnabaris	Zhu Sha 朱砂	sweet cold toxic	HT	avoid overdose and prolonged use
Rx Polygalae	Yuan Zhi 遠志	pungent bitter sl.warm	HT, LU	contra gastric ulcer, gastritis

MAJOR ACTIONS: NOURISH HEART, CALM SPIRIT

secondary actions	symptoms/conditions	dose (g)
1.Lubricate Intestines 2.Promote bowel movement	1.Yin & Blood Def.- constipation	9-18
1.Invigorate Blood 2.Resolve abscess	1.Qi Stagn. due to emotional factors 2.traumas 3.lung abscess	Fl-3-9 Cx-9-15
1.Dispel Wind 2.Invigorate Collaterals	1.Bi syndrome	9-30
1.Strengthen LIV 2.Astringe perspiration	1.HT & LIV Yin Def. 2.spontaneous & night sweats	9-18
1.Relieve convulsions 2.Detoxify	1.epilepsy 2.skin lesions	0.3-1
1.Remove Phlegm 2.Clear Orifices 3.Resolve abscess	1.Phlegm misting the HT 2.any abscess	3-9

CHAPTER 15

DIURETIC HERBS

DEFINITION: Any herb that promotes and eases urination, reduces swelling and excretes Dampness falls into this category.

GENERALIZATION: This category of diuretics are classified into 3 subcategories according to their individual major actions. They are 1) Antihydropic Diuretic 2) Urinary Soothing Diuretic and 3) Jaundice Relieving Diuretic herbs.

Most herbs tend to be bland in taste and enter the Bladder Channel.
They are used in edema, difficult urination, Wind Damp (Bi) arthritic conditions, jaundice, Damp Heat conditions, diarrhea, skin lesions caused by Damp and Heat pathogens.

Since most of the diuretic herbs treat in a symptomatic fashion, one must combine other herbs to take care of the underlying cause.

CAUTIONS AND CONTRAINDICATIONS: Generally speaking, since diuretics promote excretion of water from the body, they should be used with caution in conditions with Yin and Body Fluid Deficiency.

PHARMACOLOGICAL ACTIONS: Besides promoting diuresis, these herbs also have been found to cause contraction of gall bladder, increase bile secretion, and lower blood pressure in lab experiments. Some are also antibiotic and antifungal in action.

SECTION ONE

ANTIHYDROPIC DIURETIC HERBS

DEFINITION: Herbs that regulate water metabolism and relieve edema are called Antihydropic diuretics.

GENERALIZATION: These herbs promote urination to excrete Dampness and to relieve swelling. Some are even used in arthritic (wind damp) conditions. Because most of the herbs treat in a symptomatic fashion, one must remove the underlying cause in able to properly cure the condition. This is especially true in cases of Deficiency such as Qi Deficiency and Yang Deficiency of various organs whereby administering Tonic herbs in conjunction with diuretic herbs will achieve a much better result.

SYMPTOMATOLOGY: edema, heaviness, scanty and difficult urination, achy muscles and joints, suppurative skin lesions, etc.

SECTION 2

URINARY SOOTHING DIURETIC HERBS

DEFINITION: Any herb that promotes urination, clears Heat and relieves urinary discomfort falls into this category.

GENERALIZATION: Herbs in this category tend to be cooling and they all enter the Bladder Channel. They are mainly used, as their name implies, in urinary disorders or in Chinese medical terms, Lin Syndromes.
  Although some herbs are especially used for a particular Lin Syndrome, one must always combine other appropriate herbs to care for the underlying cause and to enhance the effect. In cases of dribbling and frequent urination due to weakness, it is not advisable to administer Diuretic herbs to further weaken the condition, instead, Tonics are recommended.

SYMPTOMATOLOGY: The Lin Syndromes in Chinese Medicine encompass all urinary disorders. Each is characteristic in their symptomatology and treatment principle. On the next page is table 12 which differentiates the various Lin Syndromes.

CAUTIONS AND CONTRAINDICATIONS: Since Urinary Soothing herbs are draining in nature, they are not suitable for use in Deficiency conditions, seminal emission and enuresis.

TABLE 12 - LIN SYNDROMES

CONDITION	SIGNS & SYMPTOMS	TX PRINCIPLE
STONE LIN	scanty difficult urination occasional gravel in urine sometimes sudden obstruction of urine with excruciating pain in back, abdomen and urethra with bloody urine P-rapid or choppy	Ease urination Expel DampHeat Dissolve stone
BLOOD LIN	**Excess Heat** reddish urine with burning pain and urgency, T-thin, yellow coat, P-full & rapid	Clear Heat Cool the Blood
	Deficient Heat chronic pale red urination slight pain, T-red, no coat P-rapid & thready	Nourish Yin Clear Heat
QI LIN	**Qi Stagnation** painful uneasy urinary flow pain and distention in lower abdomen, emotionally unstable P-wiry and deep	Regulate Qi Remove Stag.
	Prolapse of Qi pale face, sinking sensation in lower abdomen, painful urine with urgency, dribbling T-pale, P-weak	Tonify Qi Support the Middle Jiao
TURBID LIN	painful & burning urination urine cloudy & thick with sticky substance, T-red, greasy coat, P-rapid, thready	Excrete Damp-Heat Clear Bladder
EXHAUSTION LIN	chronic frequent incomplete urine, dribbling, aggravated by over strain and fatigue low back pain, paleness, shortness of breath, P-weak	Tonify Kidney Benefit Spleen

SECTION 3

JAUNDICE RELIEVING DIURETIC HERBS

DEFINITION: Herbs that excrete Dampness, benefit Gall Bladder & relieve jaundice are called Jaundice Relieving Diuretic herbs.

GENERALIZATION: These herbs have strong actions in dispelling Dampness from the body, especially from the Gall Bladder, which is the cause of abnormal yellow skin pigmentation via the urine. According to Chinese Medicine, the abnormal yellowing of the skin is due to two causes, mainly that of Damp Heat type and Damp Cold type. They are respectively termed Yang Jaundice and Yin Jaundice.

The herbs in this category are used primarily for Yang Jaundice or the Damp Heat type Jaundice. However, when properly combined with Interior Warming herbs, they can also be used for the Damp Cold type or Yin Jaundice.

During the treatment of jaundice, if the Damp factor is excessive, one may add Aromatic Damp Resolving herbs. Similarly, if the Heat factor becomes overwhelming, combination with Heat Clearing herbs should enhance the effect.

SYMPTOMATOLOGY: Below, table 13 lists the different types of jaundice.

TABLE 13 - DIFFERENTIATION OF JAUNDICE

CONDITION	SIGNS & SYMPTOMS	COMBINE WITH
YANG JAUNDICE	**Heat predominance** Bright yellow pigmentation of the skin and eyes, fever thirst, scanty yellow urine constipation, abd. fullness nausea, vomit, irritability T-yellow and greasy coat P-wiry and rapid	Clear Heat and Detoxify herbs Purgative herbs
	Damp predominance yellow pigmentation of body not as bright as in Heat predominant type, heaviness chest and stomach fullness and pressure, poor appetite abdominal distention, loose stool, T-thick greasy slight yellow coat, P-slippery	Aromatic Damp Resolving herb Clear Heat and Detoxify herbs
YIN JAUNDICE	Dull yellowing of the skin poor appetite, epigastric & abdominal distention, loose stool, fear of cold, fatigue T-pale, greasy coat P-slow and deep	Spleen Tonic & Interior Warming herbs

CATEGORY: ANTIHYDROPIC DIURETIC HERBS

pharmaceutical name	pin-yin	taste & energy	meridians	comments
Poria Cocos	Fu Ling 茯苓	sweet bland neutral	HT, LU SP, UB	
Grifolia	Zhu Ling 豬苓	"	KID, UB	stronger diuretic than Poria
Rz Alismatis	Ze Xie 澤瀉	sweet bland cold	"	
Sm Coicis	Yi Yi Ren 薏苡仁	sweet bland sl.cold	SP, ST LU, LI	
Sm Benincasae	Dong Gua Zi 冬瓜子	sweet sl.cold	LU, ST SI	
Rx Stephaniae	Fang Ji 防己	bitter pungent cold	LU, SP UB	
Stylus Zeae	Yu Mi Xu 玉米鬚	sweet neutral	UB, LIV GB	

CATEGORY: URINARY SOOTHING DIURETIC HERBS

pharmaceutical name	pin-yin	taste & energy	meridian	comments
Talcum	Hua Shi Fen 滑石粉	sweet cold	ST, UB	
Cx Zingiberis	Sheng Jiang Pi 生姜皮	pungent, cool		

106

MAJOR ACTIONS: PROMOTE DIURESIS, REDUCE SWELLING

secondary actions	symptoms/conditions	dose (g)
1.Strengthen SP 2.Calm Spirit	1.SP Def. Dampness 2.insomnia 3.irritability	6-18
none		6-18
1.Clear Damp Heat of Lower Jiao	1.Lower Jiao Heat	3-12
1.Remove Bi 2.Clear Heat, Remove Pus 3.Strengthen SP 4.Stop diarrhea	1.Bi syndrome 2.LU & ST Heat 3.lung abscess 4.SP Def. diarrhea	9-30
1.Clear Heat 2.Resolve Phlegm 3.Reduce Pus	1.LU Heat cough 2.LU & intest. abscess 3.leukorrhea	9-15
1.Dispel Wind Damp 2.Stop pain	1.Bi syndrome-Heat Bi	6-12
1.Relieve jaundice 2.Reduce blood pressure 3.Stop bleeding	1.jaundice 2.high blood pressure 3.epistaxis 4.diabetes	15-60

MAJOR ACTION: PROMOTE DIURESIS, RELIEVE URINARY DISCOMFORT

secondary actions	symptoms/conditions	dose (g)
1.Clear Summer Heat	1.Summer Heat & Damp 2.ext. for skin disease	6-18
1.Promotes diuresis, reduces swelling	1.Edema, dysuria	3-6g

Medulla Junci	Deng Xin Cao 燈心草	"	HT, SI SP	
Sm Malvae	Dong Kui Zi 冬葵子	sweet cold	LI, SI	
Sm Plantaginis	Che Qian Zi 車前子	sweet sl.cold	LU, SI UB, KID LIV	
Fr Kochiae	Di Fu Zi 地膚子	sweet bitter cold	UB	
Hb Polygoni Avicularis	Bian Xu 萹蓄	bitter cool	"	
Hb Pyrrosiae	Shi Wei 石葦	bitter cool	LU, UB	
Hb Dianthi	Qu Mai 瞿麥	bitter cold	HT, SI UB	contra. pregnant
Caulis Akebiae	Mu Tong 木通	"	"	
Rx Dioscoreae Bishie	Bi Xie 萆薢	bitter sl.cold	LIV, ST	

1.Clear HT Fire	1.HT Fire	6-15
1.Aid lactation 2.Lubricate intestines	1.lactostasis 2.constiption	9-15
1.Clear Heat, Brighten eyes 2.Stop cough	1.LIV Heat 2.LU Heat cough	3-12

1.Eliminate Damp Heat
2.Stop itching
	1.pruritis,urticaria
	  eczema
	2.nephritis,acute inf.
	  of urinary system
		6-15

1.Soothe urination
2.Anti-helminthic
3.Stop itching
	1.difficult,painful,
	  burning or bloody
	  urination
	2.itching,eczema,ext.-
	  trichomonas
		9-15

1.Soothe urination 2.Cool Blood, Stop bleeding 3.Stop cough, Resolve Phlegm	1.Lin Syndrome, esp. blood/stone Lin 2.LU Heat cough	9-15
1.Eliminate Damp Heat		6-12
1.Clear Heat 2.Aid lactation 3.Aid menstruation	1.HT Fire 2.lactostasis 3.amenorrhea 4.Bi syndrome-Heat Bi	3-9
1.Clear Turbid Damp 2.Remove Wind Damp	1.chylouria,leukorrhea 2.Bi syndrome	9-15

CATEGORY: JAUNDICE RELIEVING DIURETIC HERBS				
pharmaceutical name	pin-yin	taste & energy	meridian	comments
Hb Artemesiae Capillaris	Yin Chen Hao 茵陳蒿	bitter sl.cold	SP, ST LIV, UB	

MAJOR ACTION: DISPEL DAMPNESS, RELIEVE JAUNDICE		
scondary actions	symptoms/conditions	dose (g)
1.Clear Heat 2.Relieve jaundice	1.Damp Heat jaundice	9-15

CHAPTER 16

ANTIRHEUMATIC HERBS (WIND DAMP DISPELLING)

DEFINITION: Any herb that acts to remove Wind Damp factors from the muscles, channels and collaterals, and tendons(sinews) and bones is considered an Antirheumatic herb.

GENERALIZATION: Antirheumatic herbs can be further categorized into 3 sub-categories based upon the levels of the body. Imaging 3 levels of disease progression within the body: pathogenic Wind and Damp factors combined with Cold or Heat factors invade the body first at the 1) Superficial Muscle layer, then penetrating deeper to affect the 2) Channel layer; and over a period of time, these pathogenic factors seep slowly deeper and eventually eroding the 3) Tendon and Bone layer of the body. The pathogens can also affect more than 1 level of the body at one time.

These herbs are mostly <u>pungent</u> and beside removing Wind Damp factors, some of them also function to Disperse Cold, Activate blood circulation, Unblock Channels and Collaterals, Relax Tendons, Strengthen Bones and Tendons, and Relieve pain.

Wind Damp conditions or "Bi" syndromes as it is referred to in Chinese Medicine, are characterized by pain and disability of the joints and limbs. Below, you will find a differentiation of the "Bi" syndromes.

SYMPTOMATOLOGY: Antirheumatic or Wind Damp Dispelling herbs are used in the following conditions: Arthritis, Rheumatism, stiffness in the joints, pain and numbness of the extremities, spasms, back pain, etc. Below, table 14 shows the different types of Bi Syndromes.

TABLE 14 - DIFFERENTIATION OF "BI" SYNDROMES

CONDITION TYPE	SIGNS AND SYMPTOMS	COMBINE WITH
WIND BI (PREDOMINANCE)	MIGRATORY pains of joints and limbs, spasms	Blood Invigorating herbs
COLD BI (PREDOMINANCE)	FIXED excruciating pains of joints and limbs, worse with cold and relieved by heat	Yang Invigorating herbs Channel Warming herbs
DAMP BI (PREDOMINANCE)	DULL pain, heavy & stiff joints and limbs, local swelling, numbness	Diuretic herbs Spleen Tonic
HEAT BI (PREDOMINANCE)	BURNING pain, redness, swelling and heat sensation of joints	Heat Clearing & Antitoxin herbs

CONTRAINDICATIONS: One must exercise caution when using some of the more pungent and warming Antirheumatics in Yin and Blood Deficient conditions.

PHARMACOLOGICAL ACTIONS: These herbs have general anti-inflammatory, anti-pyretic, analgesic and vasodilatory effects.

SECTION 1

WIND DAMP DISPELLING & PAIN RELIEVING HERBS
(MUSCLE LAYER)

DEFINITION: Herbs that dispel Wind Damp factors from the muscle layer and relieve pain falls into this category.

GENERALIZATION: Although this category of herbs will focus on dispelling the pathogens from the more Superficial Muscle layer, they can also be used in deeper layers depending on the right combination of other Antirheumatic herbs. These herbs have obvious pain relieving effects and are sometimes employed just for this function.

In the beginning stages of BI syndrome, it may accompany with Exterior symptomatology. In these cases, Diaphoretic herbs must be combined to properly cure the condition.

SYMPTOMATOLOGY: Muscles aches, chills, no sweat, stiffness of neck and limbs, back and joint pains.

SECTION 2

CHANNEL INVIGORATING ANTIRHEUMATIC HERBS
(CHANNEL LAYER)

DEFINITION: Herbs that dispel Wind Damp factors from the Channel layer, promote circulation in the channels and collaterals, and relieve spasm and stiffness fall into this category.

GENERALIZATION: Herbs in this category helps to Invigorate Channels and Collaterals, Remove Blockages, Dispel Wind Damp, and to Rehabilitate disability of the joints and limbs.

Frequently, Blood Invigorating and Nourishing herbs are combined to further facilitate the circulation and lubricate the tendons.

SYMPTOMATOLOGY: One will frequently experience, as a result of Wind Damp Obstructing the channels, pain, stiffness, spasms, numbness, paralysis and disability.

SECTION 3

BONES & TENDON STRENGTHENING ANTIRHEUMATIC HERBS

DEFINITION: Herbs that dispel Wind Damp and strengthens Bones and Tendons (sinews) fall under this category.

GENERALIZATION: Herbs in this category not only dispel Wind Damp factors from the deeper level of the body, they also Tonify the bones and tendons that were the area of affection.

Wind Damp conditions or Bi syndromes which affect the body over long period of time can start to erode the tendons and bones which are governed by the Liver and the Kidneys respectively. Indirectly, the pathogens weaken the organs so that the accompanying conditions often reveal Kidney & Liver Deficiency. Therefore, along with Antirheumatic herbs in these cases, Kidney and Liver Tonic herbs are often combined with the prescription. And once the condition is relieved or under control, these Bone & Tendon Strengthening Antirheumatics can be used to prevent the recurrence of the condition.

SYMPTOMATOLOGY: The picture often paints an elderly patient suffering from arthritic conditions over long period of time with pain in the joints especially the knees and the hips, back pain, weak limbs, spasms, difficulty walking, easily fractured, calcium loss, deformities, etc. In addition to the above symptomatology, the patient probably also have weak vision, ringing in the ear, dizziness, chronic fatigue, shortness of breath, frequent urination, and a weak pulse.

CATEGORY: WIND DAMP DISPELLING & PAIN RELIEVING ANTIRHEUMATICS

pharmaceutical name	pin-yin	taste & energy	meridians	comments
Rx Clematis	Wei Ling Xian 威靈仙	pungent warm	all 12 channels	
Rx Gentianae Macrophyllae	Qin Jiao 秦艽(艽)	bitter pungent warm	LIV	
Fr Xanthii	Cang Er Zi 蒼耳子	"	LU	
Rx Angelica Tuhuo	Du Huo 獨活	pungent bitter	KID, UB	esp. good for lower body
Cx Erythrinae	Hai Tong Pi 海桐皮	pungent bitter sl.cold	LIV, SP KID	contra anemia

CATEGORY: CHANNEL INVIGORATING ANTIRHEUMATICS

pharmaceutical name	pin-yin	taste & energy	meridian	comments
Rx Aconiti Kusnezoffii	Zhi Cao Wu 制草烏	pungent bitter hot toxic	HT, LIV SP	precook 2 hrs to reduce toxicity contra pregnant extremely toxic- use cautiously
Hb Siegesbeckiae	Xi Xian Cao 豨簽草	pungent bitter sl.cold	LIV, HT	
Rx Aconiti Carmichaeli	Chuan Wu (raw Fu Zi) 川烏	pungent bitter, hot and toxic	Liv, Ht, Sp	contra pregnancy, heat & Yin Def cond

MAJOR ACTIONS: DISPEL WIND & DAMP, RELIEVE PAIN		
secondary actions	symptoms/conditions	dose (g)
1.Clear channels 2.Stop pain	1.cook with sugar, wine and vinegar to dissolve bones stuck in throat	3-12
1.Clear Deficient Heat 2.Relieve jaundice	1."Steaming Bone" sens. due to Def. Heat 2.Damp Heat jaundice	6-12
1.Clear nasal sinus 2.Stop pain	1.sinus problems 2.Bi pain 3.itching conditions	3-10
1.Stop pain	1.Bi syndrome 2.Wind Cold 3.toothache	3-9
1.Clear Channels, Stop pain	1.Bi pain, lumbago, pain & spasms of 2.chronic eczema	3-12

MAJOR ACTION: DISPEL WIND & DAMP, INVIGORATE CHANNELS, STOP SPASMS		
secondary actions	symptoms/conditions	dose (g)
1.Warm Channels, Stop pain	1.Cold Bi-severe pain hernia,migrane,trauma ext-tumors	3-9
1.Clear Channels & Collaterals 2.Detoxify		10-15
1.Warms channels, stops pain 2.Expels wind, damp and cold	1.Anti-neoplastic 2.Bi syndrome 3.Hernia 4.Internal cold/pain 5.Liver cancer	3-9g boil over 1 hr

pharmaceutical name	pin-yin	taste & energy	meridian	comments
Fr Chaenomelis Lagenariae	Mu Gua 木瓜	sour warm	LIV, SP	
Rm Mori	Sang Zhi 桑枝	bitter neutral	LIV	

CATEGORY: BONES & TENDON STRENGTHENING ANTIRHEUMATICS				
pharmaceutical name	pin-yin	taste & energy	meridian	comments
Cx Acanthopanacis	Wu Jia Pi 五加皮	pungent warm	LIV, KID	
Rx dipsaci	Xu Duan 續斷	pungent bitter sl.warm	LIV, KID	with wine to tonify with salt to descend
Os Tigris	Hu Gu 虎骨	pungent sweet warm	LIV, KID	take in powder or pill form
Agkistrodon	Bai Hua She 白花蛇	sweet salty warm toxic	"	caution Blood Def.

1.Activate Channels, Relax tendons 2.Harmonize St, Aid digestion 3.Resolve Damp	1.spasms, difficulty walking 2.Summer Heat & Damp 3.indigestion	6-12
1.Clear Channels	1.Bi of extremities	9-15

MAJOR ACTION: **DISPEL WIND & DAMP, STRENGTHEN BONES & TENDONS**

secondary actions	symptoms/conditions	dose (g)
1.Strengthen Bones & Tendons	1.Deficient Bi syndrome	9-15
1.Strengthen LIV and KID 2.Heal fractured bones 3.Stop bleeding, Prevent miscarrage	1.Bi pain in back and joints 2.fractures, traumas 3.functional uterine bleeding, threatened abortion	9-15
1.Strengthen Bones and Tendons 2.Relieve Spasms	1.Bi pain 2.infantile convulsion, tetanus	2-5
1.Stop pain 2.Strengthen Bones & Tendons	1.Def. Bi syndrome	10-15

CHAPTER 17

HEMOSTATIC HERBS

DEFINITION: Herbs that stop bleeding are called Hemostatic herbs.

GENERALIZATION: Hemostatic herbs can be further classified into 4 subcategories based on their actions. Bleeding, according to Chinese Medicine has various causes, thus, the treatment priciple differs accordingly. Some of the main causes are trauma, injuries, Heat in the Blood, Blood Stagnation, Cold Obstruction of the Channels, and Spleen Deficiency.

These herbs are classified into 1) Astringent Hemostatic 2) Blood Cooling Hemostatic 3) Unobstructing Hemostatic and 4) Channel Warming Hemostatic herbs.

In general, most Hemostatic herbs become enhanced in action when <u>charred</u> or carbonized into ashes. In his book of Grand Materia Medica, Dr. <u>Li Shi Zhen</u> stated that "when the Red [blood] sees the Black [ashes], it will cease to flow." Just like in the Five Element theory, the water reigns control over the fire. However, it is a general rule and there is always exceptions in that few herbs actually experience decrease in their hemostatic function when charred.

Bleeding can be managed under normal conditions and proper care, but in case of massive bleeding one must act quickly to stop bleeding and reinforce the Yuan (original) Qi to prevent shock.

SYMPTOMATOLOGY: Bleeding can occur anywhere in the body where there are vasculature. One can bleed internally or externally, and by carefully observing the signs and symptoms, bleeding can usually be stopped when treated properly. Most often, one can obviously see bleeding occurring from the orifices like the openings of the body such as nose bleed, eyes bleed, coughing up blood, vomiting of blood, blood in the urine, blood in the stools, abnormal uterine bleeding, bruising under the skin, and so forth.

PHARMACOLOGICAL ACTIONS: Administering of these herbs have been observed to increase platelet counts and have peripheral vasoconstriction effects while increasing blood flow in the coronary arteries. Many also have anti-inflammatory, and antibiotic functions.

SECTION ONE

ASTRINGENT HEMOSTATIC HERBS

DEFINITION: Herbs that stops bleeding by means of astringing the vessels and the tissues fall into this category.

GENERALIZATION: This category of herbs stops bleeding by their <u>astringent</u> property. They are used in many different types of bleeding, especially those due to Deficiency conditions or simple external cuts. Most can be charred in appropriate occasions to enhance the hemostatic effect.

CONTRAINDICATIONS: These herbs are not suitable for use in Excess Heat or Blood Stagnation conditions.

SECTION TWO

BLOOD COOLING HEMOSTATIC HERBS

DEFINITION: Herbs that stop bleeding by Cooling the Heat in the blood fall into this category.

GENERALIZATION: This category of herbs are either <u>cold</u> or <u>cooling</u> in nature, and are used for bleeding as a result of Heat in the Blood. When administering Blood Cooling Hemostatics, other Blood Cooling and Yin Tonic herbs should be used as adjunct. Also, if there is obvious stagnation, one may consider employing some Blood and Qi Invigorating herbs in appropriate instances.

SYMPTOMATOLOGY: One of the many causes of bleeding is due to Heat in the Blood (Xue). Below, the symptomatology is listed in table form.

CONDITION	SIGNS AND SYMPTOMS	PATHOLOGY
HEAT IN THE XUE STAGE (blood)	high fever, delirium, insomnia, mania, coma, signs of bleeding, i.g. vomiting of blood, nose bleed, bloody stool, bruising underneath the skin, tremors & spasms P-rapid and thready, T-dark red with prickles, brown burnt coat	pathogenic Heat at the deepest level is driving blood out of vessels & invade the heart (spirit), starting to create a current (LIV Wind)

CONTRAINDICATIONS: Cooling Hemostatic herbs can sometimes cause Stagnation of Qi and Blood, therefore, in cases complicated by obstructions administer the herbs carefully and not excessively. They are also not recommended for conditions of Cold and Deficient Spleen.

122

SECTION THREE

UNOBSTRUCTING HEMOSTATIC HERBS

DEFINITION: Herbs that stop bleeding by removing Stagnations fall into this category.

GENERALIZATION: Herbs in this category act to stop bleeding by removing obstructions. One may be puzzled that if the purpose here is to stop blood from flowing out why is it then that a Stagnation needs to be removed so that bleeding can be stopped! Just visualize blood circulating in the channels and vessels and came upon a blockade which hampers the flow. With time, pressure builds and soon the blood seeps through to find another outlet or the vessel simply bursts, eventually lead to bleeding. This blockade can be caused by various factors such as trumatic injuries, emotional damage and cold stagnation. Therefore, frequently they are aided with Qi and Blood Invigorating herbs to quickly resolve the obstruction and stop the bleeding.

CAUTIONS AND CONTRAINDICATIONS: Some herbs are contraindicated in pregnancy.

SECTION FOUR

CHANNEL WARMING HEMOSTATIC HERBS

DEFINITION: Herbs that stop bleeding by means of Warming the channels and dispelling the Coldness fall into this category.

GENERALIZATION: These herbs are _warm_ in nature. They act to stop bleeding by Warming the Channels, dispelling Cold and restoring normal blood flow.
     Channel Warming Hemostatic herbs are used primarily for bleeding due to Deficiency and Coldness. When the Yang Qi of the body is weak (mainly that of the spleen), it cannot properly contain and guide the blood in the Channels and vessels, thus the blood extravasates. Or when the Cold constricts the passage way, it causes bleeding which can be mended by Warming the passage way and Resolving the obstruction.
     Most of the time, Yang Tonic herbs are utilized as an adjunct.

CAUTIONS AND CONTRAINDICATIONS: Because these herbs are warm, they are contraindicated in bleeding due to Blood Heat and Yin Deficiency patients.

CATEGORY: ASTRINGENT HEMOSTATIC HERBS

pharmaceutical name	pin-yin	taste & energy	meridians	comments
Rz Bletillae	Bai Ji 白芨	bitter sweet astring sl.cold	LIV, LU ST	contra. with Rx Aconiti
Hb Agrimoniae	Xian He Cao 仙鶴草	bitter astring neutral	LU, LIV SP	
Crinis Carbino-satus	Xue Yu Tan 血餘炭	bitter neutral	"	use in powder form

CATEGORY: BLOOD COOLING HEMOSTATIC HERBS

pharmaceutical name	pin-yin	taste & energy	meridian	comments
Rx Sanguisorbae	Di Yu 地榆	bitter sour sl.cold	LIV, ST LI	
Fl Sophorae	Huai Hua 槐花	bitter sl.cold	LIV, LI	
Caucumen Biotae	Ce Bai Ye 側柏葉	bitter astring	LIV, LU LI	
Hb Cirsii Segeti (C. Japonici)	Da Ji 大薊	sweet	HT, LIV cold	

MAJOR ACTIONS: ASTRINGE & STOP BLEEDING

secondary actions	symptoms/conditions	dose (g)
1.Astringent-hemostatic 2.Aid wound healing	1.hemorrhage cond.-esp of LU, ST 2.chronic wounds	5-15
1.Astringent-hemostatic 2.Detoxify 3.Anti-helminthic	1.hemorrhage 2.dysentery 3.malaria 4.trichomonis vaginitis	10-15
1.Remove Stagnation-hemostatic 2.Nourish Yin, Ease urination 3.astrigent-hemostatic	1.functional uterine bleeding, hematuria 2.dysuria	1.5-3

MAJOR ACTION: COOL THE BLOOD, STOP BLEEDING

secondary actions	symptoms/conditions	dose (g)
1.Cool Blood-hemostatic 2.Consolidate Fluids 3.Detoxify	1.Blood Heat-esp. Lower Jiao 2.burns, skin disease	10-15
1.Cool Blood-hemostatic 2.Lower blood pressure	1.Blood Heat-esp hema-feces, hemorrhoids 2.hypertension	8-16
1.Cool Blood-hemostatic 2.Stop cough	1.Blood Heat hemorrhage 2.LU Heat cough 3.burns	10-15
1.Cool Blood-hemostatic 2.Reduce swelling	1.Blood Heat hemorrhage 2.skin disease	10-15

CATEGORY: UNOBSTRUCTING HEMOSTATIC HERBS

pharmaceutical name	pin-yin	taste & energy	meridian	comments
Rx Pseudoginseng	San Qi 三七	sweet sl.bitr warm	LIV, ST	contra. pregnant
Pollen Typhae	Pu Huang 蒲黄	sweet neutral	LIV, HT	

CATEGORY: CHANNEL WARMING HEMOSTATIC HERBS

pharmaceutical name	pin-yin	taste & energy	meridian	comments
Fm Artemisiae	Ai Ye 艾葉	bitter pungent warm	LIV, SP KID	

MAJOR ACTION: REMOVE OBSTRUCTION, STOP BLEEDING		
secondary actions	symptoms/conditions	dose (g)
1. Remove Stagnation-hemostatic 2. Reduce swelling, Stop pain	1. hemorrhage due to Stagnation 2. trauma 3. coronary heart disease	2-6
1. Invigorate Blood flow 2. Carbonized-hemostatic 3. Ease urination	1. Blood Stagnation ie: dysmenorrhea	5-10

MAJOR ACTION: WARM UP CHANNELS, STOP BLEEDING		
secondary actions	symptoms/conditions	dose (g)
1. Warm Channels-hemostatic 2. Disperse Cold, Stop pain	1. Def. Cold bleeding- ie: excess menses 2. Cold Stagnation 3. ext-skin disease	3-9

CHAPTER 18

BLOOD INVIGORATING HERBS

DEFINITION: Herbs that facilitate blood flow and remove obstructions are called Blood Invigorating herbs.

GENERALIZATION: Disease arises when there is a blockage of Qi, and since Blood depends on Qi for movement and Qi needs nourishment from Blood to function, one can readily see that Stagnation of Blood is intimately associated with Stagnation of Qi and vice versa.

Herbs in this category are mostly <u>pungent</u>. They tend to enter the <u>Liver channel</u> which promotes smooth flow of Qi and stores blood at night and the <u>Heart channel</u> because the heart distributes blood through out the body. Blood Invigorating herbs have, as a result, secondary actions such as relieve pain, induce labor, reduce swelling and disperse hardenings.

There are many causes of Blood Stagnation. Examples include Cold Obstruction, Qi Stagnation, traumas, emotional injury, Yang Deficiency, and etc. Because of the many different causes, one must combine other appropriate herbs when treating.

SYMPTOMATOLOGY: The most obvious symptom of stagnation is PAIN. In Blood Stagnation the pain is sharp and fixed, whereas in Qi Stagnation the pain is dull, intermittent and non-stationary. Blood Stagnation in the body can cause a wide range of conditions such as amenorrhea, dysmenorrhea, puerpleral pain, tumors, abdominal masses, Bi syndrome, coronary angina and others. On the other hand, it can also be the result of external injury and traumas.

CAUTIONS AND CONTRAINDICATIONS: Because Blood Invigorating herbs have abortive function, they are contraindicated in pregnancy and excessive menstruation.

PHARMACOLOGICAL ACTIONS: Most of these herbs have been shown to have vasodilatory, antihypertensive and analgesic effects

CATEGORY: BLOOD INVIGORATING HERBS				
pharmaceutical name	pin-yin	taste & energy	meridians	comments
Rz Curcuma Longae	Jiang Huang 姜黃	pungent bitter warm	LIV, SP	contra. pregnant
Rz Zedoariae	(Pong) Er Zhu 莪茂	"	"	contra. pregnant
Rz Corydalis	Yan Hu Suo 延胡索	"	"	use in powder form contra. pregnant
Gummi Olibanum	Ru Xiang 乳香	"	HT, LIV SP	contra. pregnant
Rz Ligustici Wallichi	Chuan Xiong 川芎	pungent warm	LIV, GB P	contra. Yin Def.- Heat/Exuberance of LIV Yang
Fl Carthami	Hong Hua 紅花	pungent sl.warm	LIV, HT	contra. pregnant or excess menses
Hb Lycopi	Ze Lan 澤蘭	pungent bitter sl.warm	LIV, SP	
Fr Liquidamberis	Lu Lu Tong 路路通	pungent bitter neutral	LIV, ST UB	contra. pregnant
Rz Scirbii (Sparganii)	San Ling (San Leng) 三棱	"	LIV, SP	contra. pregnant or excess menses

MAJOR ACTIONS: INVIGORATE BLOOD, REMOVE STAGNATION

secondary actions	symptoms/conditions	dose (g)

1. Regulate menstruation
   Stop pain
	1. LIV Qi Stagnation-
	   dysmenorrhea
	2. traumas
		3-9

1. Anti-tumor 2. Invigorate Qi, Stop pain	1. carcinoma, tumor growth 2. food retention	3-9
1. Invigorate Qi flow 2. Stop pain	1. Blood/Qi Stagnation- causing pain	1.5-3

1. Stop pain
2. Reduce swelling,
   Aid wound healing
	1. Stagnation-pain
	2. chronic suppurative
	   skin lesions
		3-9

1. Invigorate Qi & Blood 2. Dispel wind 3. Stop pain	1. Blood Stagnation 2. headaches	3-9
1. Invigorate Blood, Remove Stagn. 2. Regulate menstruation 3. Induce labor	1. traumas, tumors 2. menstrual problems	3-9

1. Invigorate Blood, Promote
   menses
2. Promote Diuresis
	1. irreg. menses, post-
	   partum abd. pain,
	   dysmenorrhea
	2. traumas
	3. edema, incontinence
		6-10

1. Dispel Wind Damp 2. Invigorate Channels 3. Diuretic 4. Remove lactostasis	1. Bi syndrome 2. edema, dysuria 3. lactostasis	3-10
1. Invigorate Qi, Stop pain	1. severe Stagnations 2. food retention	3-9

Sm Persicae	Tao Ren 桃仁	"	LIV, LU LI	contra. pregnant or hemoptysis
Commiphora Myrrha	Muo Yao (Mo Yao) 没藥	bitter neutral	LIV, HT SP	contra. pregnant
Rx Curcumae	Yu Jin 鬱金	pungent bitter cold	HT, LIV GB	
Hb Leonuri	Yi Mu Cao 益母草	pungent bitter sl.cold	LIV, HT UB	contra. pregnant
Hb Patriniae	Bai Jiang Cao 敗醬草	"	LIV, ST LI	
Rx Salviae	Dan Shen 丹參	bitter sl.cold	HT, P LIV	contra with Rx Aconiti
Rx Rubiae	Qian Cao 茜草	bitter cold	HT, LIV	charred to stop bleeding
Rx Achyranthis	Niu Xi 牛膝	bitter sour neutral	LIV, KID	contra pregnant or excess menses
Pyritum	Zi Ren Tong 自然銅	pungent neutral	LIV	use in powder or pill form

132

1.Lubricate intestines 2.Stop cough, dyspnea	1.constipation 2.cough, dyspnea	6-10

1.Stop pain
2.Reduce swelling,
  Aid wound healing
	1.Stagnation-pain
	2.chronic suppurative
	  skin lesions
		3-9

1.Invigorate Qi flow 2.Cool Blood, Clear Heat 3.Relieve jaundice	1.LIV Qi Stagnation 2.Blood Heat-hemorrhage 3.jaundice	3-9
1.Invigorate Blood, Remove Stagnation 2.Ease urination 3.Detoxify	1.menstrual problems 2.dysuria 3.skin disease	10-30

1.Remove Blood Stagnation,
  Relieve pain
2.Detoxify, Resolve abscess
	1.post partum pain,
	  dysmenorrhea, endo-
	  metritis
	2.intestinal abscess
	3.acute appendicitis,
	  carbuncles
		6-15

1.Invigorate Blood, Remove Stagnation 2.Cool Blood, Reduce swelling 3.Calm the Spirit	1.Blood Stagnation 2.hepatomegaly 3.Ying Stage Heat	3-15

1.Invigorate Blood,
  Remove Stagnation
2.Clear Heat, Stop bleeding
3.Stop cough, Expel Phlegm
	1.splenomegaly, hepato-
	  megaly, ext traumas
	2.functional uterine
	  bleeding
	3.chronic bronchitis
		10-15

1.Invigorate Blood, Remove Stagn. 2.Tonify LIV & KID 3.Ease urination 4.Descend Blood Heat	1.menstrual problems 2.weak back & joints 3.dysuria 4.Upper Jiao Blood Heat	6-15
1.Stop pain 2.Aid bone healing	1.fractures	.3-.5

Lignum Sappan	Su Mu 蘇木	"	"	contra pregnant
Rx Paeoniae Rubra	Chi Shao 赤芍	bitter sour sl.cold	LIV, SP	caution Blood Def.
Faeces Trogopterorum	Wu Ling Zhi 五靈脂	bitter sweet warm	"	contra with Rx Ginseng caution pregnant
Fl Rosae Chinensis	Yue Ji Hua 月季花	sweet sl.warm	LIV	contra pregnant or SP/ST Deficiency
Succinum	Hu Po 琥珀	sweet neutral	LIV, HT SI, UB	powder/pill form
Resina Draconis	Xue Jie 血竭	sweet salty neutral	P, LIV	use in powder form
Squama Manitis	Chuan Shan Jia 穿山甲	salty sl.cold	LIV, ST	use in powder form
Sm Vaccariae	Wang Bu Liu Xing 王不留行	pungent sweet neutral	"	contra pregnant
Mylabris	Ban Zi (Ban Mao) 斑蝥	pungent warm toxic	"	contra pregnant powder/pill form

1.Reduce swelling, Stop pain	1.traumas	3–10

1.Remove Blood Stagnation, Reduce swelling, Stop pain
2.Clear Heat, Cool Blood
	1.amenorrhea,menor-
	   rhalgia
	2.acute inflam. with
	   redness & swelling
	3.epistaxis,rash,hemat-
	   emesis,febrile disease
		6–15

1.Remove Blood Stagnation, Stop
   pain
	1.amenorrhea,abd.pain
	   dysmenorrhea,lochia
	   retention
	2.coronary heart disease
	   angina pectoris
		3–9

1.Invigorate Blood, Regulate
   menstruation
2.Reduce swelling
	1.dysmenorrhea,
	   amenorrhea
	2.scrofula, etc.
		5–8

1.Invigorate Blood, Remove
   Stagnation
2.Calm Spirit
3.Promote Diuresis, Reduce
   swelling
	1.HT Blood Def.amenorr-
	2.Internal Wind
	3.acute UTI,UB stones
	4.coronary heart disease
		1.5–3

1.Invigorate Blood, Remove
   Stagnation
2.Stop bleeding, Resolve pain
3.Aid wound healing
	1.trauma, bleeding due
	   to blood Stagnation
	2.chronic wounds not
	   healing
		1–1.5

1.Regulate menses, Aid lactation 2.Ext-Hemostatic 3.Resolve pus	1.lactostasis 2.tumors, lymphoadeno- pathy 3.skin disease	1–1.5
1.Invigorate Blood, Regulate menstruation 2.Aid lactation	1.amenorrhea 2.lactostasis 3.dysuria	4–10
1.Invigorate Blood 2.Detoxify, Disperse Hardening 3.Aid wound healing	1.carcinoma of viscera 2.swollen lymph glands 3.psoriasis	.03–.06

135

Concha Arecae	Wa Leng Zi 瓦楞子	salty neutral	LIV, ST LU	powdered
Rx Cyathulae officinalis	Chuan Niu Xi 川牛膝	sweet, bitter, neutral	Liv, Kid	Contra in pregnancy, seminal emission

1.Resolve Phlegm 2.Remove Stagnation 3.Soften Hardenings	1.scrofula 2.tumors 3.gastric ulcer	6-30 (powder- use 3-9)
1.Expels Wind Damp 2.Activates Channels	1.Invigorate Blood, remove stagnation 2.Bi Syndrome, esp. of lower limbs 3.Amenorrhea, Abd. tumors	4.5-9g

CHAPTER 19

TONIC HERBS

DEFINITION: Herbs that tonify body deficiencies and strengthen the Antipathogenic Qi are called Tonic herbs.

GENERALIZATION: These herbs are called Tonic herbs because they replenish insufficiencies of all aspects of the body, including Qi, blood, body fluid, Yin, Yang, organs, musculoskeletal degeneration, reproductive weakness and so forth. For easier application, they are classified into four subcategories, mainly herbs that tonify the Yin, Yang, Qi and blood.

Because of the interdependence between the Yin and Yang, Qi and Blood, a Deficient condition can involve more then one aspect or it can lead to Deficiency in another area. For instance, Qi Deficiency often leads to Yang Deficiency, and Yang Deficiency often includes Qi Deficiency; this is a reflection of functional weakness. On the other hand, Deficiency in the Blood will frequently result in Deficiency of the Yin, and Yin Deficiency may include Blood Deficiency; this will result in emaciation of the material body. Therefore, one must be considerate of all factors involved and apply appropriate synergistic herbs.

When a Deficient condition is complicated with pathogens, one may choose proper methods to expel the pathogens in addition to administering the Tonic herbs. This will vary according to the nature, strength and location of the pathogen.

Tonic herbs, in general, tend to be <u>sweet</u>, rich and hard to digest and absorb. They should be boiled longer than usual to fully extract their essence. In case of Stomach/Spleen Deficiency, one must strengthen the digestive system or else it may become a waste of effort when the patient fails to properly assimilate the Tonics. Measures also must be taken to protect the Stomach and Spleen, such as adding Qi Regulating/Carminative herbs to prevent "clogging" of the system, and administering herbs in pill form to gradually Tonify and avoid weakening of the digestion from long term intake of herbal tea.

A word of caution to those healthy individuals who wish to further strengthen themselves by taking Tonic herbs unnecessarily will find themselves worsen by it. Tonics are used only in cases of Defiency, when there is no deficiency, it can disrupt the balance of Yin and Yang, ultimately leading to disease.

SECTION ONE

QI TONIC HERBS

DEFINITION: Herbs that Tonify the Qi are called Qi Tonic herbs.

GENERALIZATION: These Qi Tonic herbs mainly work on the Lungs, Heart, Spleen and the Kidneys. Most of them are sweet and enter those organs described above. When the Qi is weak, the body will cease to function properly. Everything becomes sluggish. Sometimes the body fails to keep vital substances within or in place, leading to prolapse of organs, spontaneous sweating and emission, chronic diarrhea and so on. Please see below for a more complete description of the symptomatology.

SYMPTOMATOLOGY: When the Lung is affected, it causes shortness of breath, lethargy, feeble voice, and spontaneous sweating; when the Spleen is affected, one may see lack of appetite, emaciation, chronic diarrhea, prolapse of organs, easily bruised or bleed and anemia; when the Heart is affected, it may result in palpitations, heart pain and a weak pulse; and when the Kidney becomes weakened, frequent urination, premature ejaculation and seminal emission and weak lower back and knees may be experienced.

PHARMACOLOGICAL ACTIONS: In lab experiments, it has been observed that Qi Tonic herbs generally have stimulating action on the central nervous system. Increase in endurance (as measured by swimming time) was also noted.

SECTION TWO

YANG TONIC HERBS

"An expert at tonifying Yang always seeks the Yang from the Yin, when the Yang is assisted by the Yin, its wonders can never be exhausted."
                                                    - Zhong Jing Yue

DEFINITION: Herbs that strengthen the Yang are called Yang Tonics.

GENERALIZATION: Most of these herbs are sweet and warm in nature and all enter the Kidney channel. Some are stronger in Warming thus they are pungent and others are salty because they act on the kidneys, the Water Element.
    These herbs Strengthen the Yang of the body, but mainly that of the kidney Yang. Because the kidney in our body supplies the original Fire and Water, this is why when the Yang is weak, anywhere in the body, we can attribute it to the Kidneys as the source of the problem. The kidneys are also responsible for Producing Marrow, Governing the Bones, Receiving the Lung Qi,

Promoting growth, development and reproduction, therefore, many of the functional problems associated with the above described such as reproductive deficiency, chronic asthma, weak and fragile bones, mental retardation and malformation in children comes from a Kidney Deficiency.

Yang Tonic herbs are frequently combined with Interior Warming and Qi Tonic herbs for maximal effect. They should also be combined with Yin tonic herbs so that the Yang has support for its growth.

SYMPTOMATOLOGY: Coldness, edema, fatigue, sore and weak back and knees, frequent urination, bed wetting, impotence, seminal emission, infertility, dizziness, ringing in ears, weak limbs, diarrhea, asthma and hampered physical growth and development in children.

CAUTIONS AND CONTRAINDICATIONS: When a Yang Deficient condition co-exists with Yin or Blood Deficiency, one must use Yang Tonics with caution so as not to further disturb the balance between Yin and Yang.

PHARMACOLOGICAL ACTIONS: These herbs have been found to have general tonic effect by increasing cardiac output, increasing blood pressure in hypotensive cases, increasing sperm production, increasing work capacity and decreasing The rate of muscle fatigue.

SECTION THREE

BLOOD TONIC HERBS

"The material blood can not be replenished [by itself], it can only be formed by the non-material Qi."

- Classics

DEFINITION: Herbs that nourish the Blood and relieve anemia conditions are referred to as Blood Tonics.

GENERALIZATION: The three organs in the body that are most intimately associated with Blood are the Heart, Liver and Spleen. The Heart circulates blood through out the body, the Liver stores the blood and the Spleen produces blood.

Blood Deficiency conditions may arise from bleeding, over exertion, Yin Deficiency and Spleen Qi weakness. The blood cannot be formed without the Qi, thus, it is of special importance to combine with Qi tonics in one's prescription.

SYMPTOMATOLOGY: Pale or sallow face, pale lips and whitish nails, dizziness, blurry vision, ringing in ears, palpitations, poor memory, delayed and scanty menstruation with pale flow, sometimes amenorrhea, pale tongue and a weak and thready pulse.

CAUTIONS AND CONTRAINDICATIONS: Blood Tonics are unusually rich and tend to obstruct the digestive functions, thus they are refrained from use in conditions of Dampness invading the Middle Jiao with diarrhea. Frequently, Spleen Tonics and Digestives are added to the prescription.

PHARMACOLOGICAL ACTIONS: Very few of the herbs have been shown to increase production of red blood cell directly.

SECTION FOUR

YIN TONIC HERBS

"An expert at nourishing Yin always seeks the Yin from the Yang, when the Yin is aided by the Yang, its source can never be depleted."
- *Zhong Jing Yue*

DEFINITION: Herbs that aid in nourishing the Yin and regenerate Body Fluids are considered Yin Tonics.

GENERALIZATION: Yin Tonic herbs tend to be a bit on the cooling side. When the Yin is Deficient, the Yang would be in relative excess, thus it can produce a condition of Heat. However, this Heat is not a real Excess Heat, rather, it is derived from not enough Water in the body to counter-balance the Fire. Thus the condition is called False Heat or Yin Deficient Heat. In this case, simply administering Yin Tonics will often suffice.
There are other conditions that may exhaust the Yin such as febrile diseases injuring the body's Yin and Fluids, in these cases, herbs such as the Antipyretic/Heat Clearing herbs should be added.

SYMPTOMATOLOGY: Thirst, dry mouth and throat, dry cough sometimes with blood, dry eyes, blurry vision, vertigo, tremors, insomnia with disturbing dreams, seminal emission, sore back and knees, low grade afternoon fever, night sweat, flushed cheeks, feverish palms and soles, rapid and thready pulse and a red tongue with slight or no coat.

CAUTIONS AND CONTRAINDICATIONS: These herbs are like Blood Tonics in that they tend to be rich and thus not appropriate for weak Spleen, dampness and diarrhea conditions.

PHARMACOLOGICAL ACTIONS: These herbs generally have a regulatory function on fluid metabolism. Some also have cardiotonic and antihypertensive effects.

CATEGORY: QI TONIC HERBS				
pharmaceutical name	pin-yin	taste & energy	meridians	comments
Rz Atractylodes Alba 白术	Bai Zhu	bitter sweet warm	SP, ST	tonic-fry anti-diarrh.-char diures/sweat-raw
Fr Zizyphi Sativae 大枣	Da Zao	sweet neutral	"	
Rx Glycyrrhizae 甘草	Gan Cao	"	HT, LU SP, ST	tonify-honey bake cont. use causes high B.P., edema
Rx Polygonati 黄精	Huang Jing	"	LU, KID SP	contra. damp cond.
Rx Dioscorreae 山药	Shan Yao	"	"	
Rx Codonopsis 党参	Dang Shen	"	SP, LU	incompat-Rx Veratri
Rx Astragali 黄芪	Huang Qi	sweet sl.warm	"	
Saccharum Granorum 饴糖	Yi Tang	"	SP, ST LU	
Rx Ginseng 人参	Ren Shen	sweet sl.bitt neutral	SP, LU HT	incompatable with Rx Veratri

MAJOR ACTIONS: TONIFY QI, STRENGTHEN MIDDLE JIAO

secondary actions	symptoms/conditions	dose (g)
1. Diuretic, Dry Damp 2. Stop sweating	1. SP Def. Damp 2. spontaneous sweating	3-12
1. Nourish Blood 2. Calm Spirit 3. Harmonize other herbs	1. chronic disease of LIV/SP 2. prevent strong herbs from injuring organs	10-30 (3-10 pieces)
1. Clear Heat, Detoxify 2. Resolve Phlegm, Stop cough 3. Harmonize 4. Stop pain	1. skin lesions 2. cough 3. HT Qi Deficiency 4. abd. pain	2-9
1. Tonify Yin 2. Moisten LU 3. Strengthen SP	1. Yin Def. of LU 2. SP Deficiency	9-30
1. Strengthen KID & LU	1. chronic cough 2. KID Qi Deficiency 3. diabetes	9-30
1. Increase RBC count	1. SP/LU Qi Def. anemia	9-15
1. Raise Yang 2. Strengthen Wei Qi 3. Aid wound healing 4. Diuretic	1. Collapse of Qi 2. spontaneous sweating 3. chronic lesions 4. Def. edema	9-15
1. Moisten LU, Stop cough	1. SP/ST Deficiency 2. LU Def. cough/dryness	30-60
1. Tonify Yuan Qi 2. Strengthen LU 3. Nourish Body Fluids 4. Calm Spirit	1. shock, collapse 2. LU Qi Deficiency 3. febrile disease 4. HT Qi Deficiency	3-9 (30 for shock)

CATEGORY: YANG TONIC HERBS

pharmaceutical name	pin-yin	taste & energy	meridians	comments
Rz Drynariae	Gu Sui Bu 骨碎補	bitter warm	LIV, KID	
Rx Dipsaci	Xu Duan 續斷	"	"	
Sm Trigonellae	Hu Lu Ba 胡蘆芭	"	"	contra. pregnant
Cornu Cervi Pantotrichum	Lu Rong 鹿茸	sweet salty warm	"	powdered and taken singly
Ext. Genitalia of Callorhinus Urs.	Hai Gou 海狗腎	"	"	
Hippocampus	Hai Ma 海馬	"	"	contra. pregnant
Sm Cuscutae	Tu Si Zi 蒐絲子	pungent sweet neutral	"	
Rx Morindae	Ba Ji Tian 巴戟天	pungent sweet sl.warm	"	
Cornu Cervi	Lu Jiao 鹿角	salty, sl.warm	Liv, Kid.	

MAJOR ACTIONS: TONIFY KIDNEY, WARM KIDNEY YANG

secondary actions	symptoms/conditions	dose (g)
1. Heal bone fracture 2. Invigorate Blood	1. dislocations & fractures 2. traumas 3. Bi syndrome	10-15
1. Tonify LIV 2. Strengthen Bones & Tendons 3. Invigorate Blood 4. Stabalize fetus	1. weak limbs 2. traumas 3. hypermotility of fetus	9-15
1. Relieve pain	1. Cold pain in testes, abd. pain, edema 2. hernia	3-9
1. Benefit Jing & Blood 2. Strengthen Bones & Tendons	1. child maldevelopment 2. uterine bleeding 3. weakness & atrophy	.5-1
1. Tonify KID Yang	1. impotence, seminal emission	3-9
1. Invigorate Blood, Remove Stagnation	1. impotence, lumbago, frequent urination 2. tumor, boils, scrofula 3. difficult labor	1-1.5
1. Benefit Jing 2. Nourish LIV 3. Brighten vision	1. infertility 2. LIV/KID Deficiency-vision loss	9-15
1. Strengthen Bones & Tendons 2. Dispel Wind-Damp	1. weak limbs 2. Bi syndrome-Def. type	6-15
1. Tonifies Kid & Liv Yang 2. Nourishs Blood, tonifies Jing 3. Removes Blood Stag.	1. Kidney Def., anemia 2. back pain, impotence 3. trauma wounds	3-15g

Cx Eucommiae 杜仲	Du Zhong	sweet warm	"	
Rz Cibotii 狗脊	Gou Ji	bitter sweet warm	"	
Hb Epimedii 淫羊藿	Yin Yang Huo	pungent warm	"	
Fr Alpiniae Oxyphyllae 益智仁	Yi Zhi Ren	"	"	
Fr Psoralaeae 補骨脂	Bu Gu Zhi	pungent bitter warm	"	
Sm Allii Tuberosi 韭菜子	Jiu Cai Zi	pungent sweet warm	KID, UB	
Cordyceps 冬蟲夏草	Dong Cong Xia Cao	sweet warm	LU, KID	powdered
Gecko 蛤蚧	Ge Jie	salty neutral	"	powdered
Hb Cistanches 肉蓯蓉	Rou Cong Rong	sweet salty warm	KID, LI	
Sm Juglandis 胡桃肉	Hu Tao Rou	sweet warm	KID, LU LI	

1.Tonify LIV 2.Strengthen Bones & Tendons 3.Lower blood pressure 4.Stabilize fetus	1.LIV/KID Deficiency 2.Def.-hypertension 3.threatened abortion	9-15
1.Dispel Wind-Damp 2.Tonify LIV 3.Strengthen low back & knees	1.chronic Bi syndrome	10-15
1.Strengthen Bones & Tendons 2.Dispel Wind-Damp 3.Stop cough & asthma	1.weak limbs 2.Def. Bi syndrome 3.KID Def. cough 4.hypertension	9-15
1.Consolidate Jing 2.Astringe urination 3.Warm SP 4.Stop diarrhea	1.seminal emission 2.frequent urination, bedwetting 3.SP Yang Def. diarrhea	3-9
1.Warm SP 2.Stop diarrhea	1.SP/KID Yang Def.- "5 o'clock diarrhea"	3-9

1.Consolidate Jing	1.impotence, seminal
	  emission,enuresis,
	  polyuria
		3-9

1.Tonify LU 2.Stop cough & asthma	1.KID/LU Def.-cough, asthma	6-15

1.Tonify LU
2.Calm Rebellious Qi, Relieve
  asthma
	1.LU/KID Def. asthma,
	  cough, short of breath
		1-1.5

1.Benefit Jing 2.Lubricate Intestines	1.constipation	9-18
1.Tonify LU 2.Lubricate Intestines	1.LU/KID Def.-cough, asthma 2.constipation	9-30

pharmaceutical name	pin-yin	taste & energy	meridians	comments
Hb Cynomori	Suo Yang 鎖陽	"	KID, LIV LI	
Sm Curculiginis	Xian Mao 仙茅	pungent warm sl.tox.	KID, LIV SP	
Placenta Hominis	Zi He che 紫河車	sweet salty warm	KID, LU HT	powdered

CATEGORY: BLOOD TONIC HERBS				
pharmaceutical name	pin-yin	taste & energy	meridians	comments
Rx Angelica Sinensis	Dang Gui 當歸	pungent sweet warm	LIV, SP HT	
Arillus Longanae	Long Yan Rou 龍眼肉	sweet warm	SP, HT	
Rx Rehmanniae (cooked)	Shu Di Huang 熟地黃	sweet sl.warm	KID, LIV HT	contra. SP Def. & diarrhea
Fr Mori	Sang Shen 桑椹	sweet sl.cold	"	
Rx Polygoni Multiflori	He Shou Wu 何首烏	sweet bitter sl.warm astring	"	tonify-prepared detox/constipation-raw
Gelatinum Asini	E Jiao 阿膠	sweet neutral	KID, LIV LU	

secondary actions	symptoms/conditions	dose (g)
1. Tonify LIV 2. Lubricate Intestines	1. weak limbs 2. constipation	9-15
1. Warm SP Yang 2. Strengthen Bones & Tendons 3. Dispel Cold-Damp	1. SP Yang Deficiency 2. Bi syndrome	3-9
1. Benifit Jing 2. Strengthen Qi 3. Nourish Blood	1. infertility 2. lactation deficiency 3. cough, short of breath	1.5-3

MAJOR ACTIONS: **TONIFY BLOOD**

secondary actions	symptoms/conditions	dose (g)
1. Regulate menstruation 2. Invigorate Blood, Stop pain 3. Lubricate Intestines	1. menstrual irreg. 2. traumas 3. constipation	3-12
1. Nourish HT & SP 2. Calm Spirit	1. HT/SP Deficiency 2. insomnia	6-12
1. Nourish Yin	1. Blood Deficiency 2. Yin Deficiency	9-30
1. Nourish Yin 2. Lubricate Intestines	1. Yin Deficiency 2. constipation 3. diabetes	15-30
1. Tonify KID & LIV 2. Benefit Jing & Blood 3. Promote B.M. 4. Detoxify	1. KID/LIV Deficiency 2. premature greying 3. constipation 4. skin lesions	9-25
1. Stop bleeding 2. Nourish Yin 3. Moisten LU	1. bleeding due to Def. 2. Yin Def. Heat 3. Lu Yin Def.	6-15

pharmaceutical name	pin-yin	taste & energy	meridians	comments
Fr Lycii	Gou Qi Zi 枸杞子	"	KID, LIV	
Rx Paeoniae Alba	Shao Yao 芍藥	bitter sour sl.cold	LIV	Incompatable with Rx Veratri

<table>
CATEGORY: YIN TONIC HERBS
</table>

pharmaceutical name	pin-yin	taste & energy	meridians	comments
Rx Glehniae	Bie Sha Shen 北沙參	sweet sl.cold	ST, LU	contra with Rx Veratri
Rz Polygonati Officinalis	Yu Zhu 玉竹	"	"	
Bulbus Lilii	Bai He 百合	"	LU, HT	
Hb Dendrobi	Shi Hu 石斛	sweet bland sl.cold	LU, ST KID	
Rx Ophiopogonis	Mai Men Dong 麥門冬	sweet sl.bitt sl.cold	LU, ST HT	
Rx Panacis	Xi Yang Shen 西洋參	sweet cold	HT, LU KID	
Rx Asparagi	Tien Men Dong 天門冬	sweet bitter cold	LU, KID	contra SP Def. & diarrhea

1. Nourish Yin 2. Benefit Jing 3. Brighten eyes	1. Yin Deficiency 2. diabetes 3. visual problems	6–15
1. Subdue LIV Yang 2. Consolidates Yin 3. Soften LIV 4. Stop pain	1. LIV Yang Rising 2. LIV Yin Def. 3. LIV Qi Stagnation 4. menstrual irreg.	9–18

MAJOR ACTIONS: NOURISH YIN

secondary action	symptoms/conditions	dose (g)
1. Moisten LU 2. Strengthen ST 3. Nourish Body Fluids	1. LU Yin Deficiency 2. ST Yin Deficiency	
1. Moisten LU 2. Strengthen ST 3. Nourish Body Fluids	1. LU Yin Deficiency 2. ST Yin Deficiency	9–30
1. Moisten LU, Stop cough 2. Clear HT, Calm Spirit	1. LU Yin Def. cough 2. Heat Disturbing HT	9–15
1. Clear Heat 2. Nourish Body Fluids 3. Strengthen ST 4. Moisten LU	1. Yin Deficiency Heat 2. ST Yin Deficiency	9–20
1. Moisten LU 2. Nourish Body Fluids 3. Harmonize ST 4. Descend Rebellious Qi	1. LU Yin Deficiency 2. vomiting, cough 3. skin lesions	6–12
1. Clear Heat 2. Nourish Body Fluids	1. LU Yin Deficiency 2. Febrile Disease – damaging Body Fluids	3–6
1. Clear False Heat 2. Moisten LU 3. Nourish KID	1. Yin Deficiency Heat 2. LU Yin Deficiency 3. KID Yin Deficiency	6–24

Fr Ligustri	Nu Zhen Zi 女貞子	sweet bitter cool	LIV, KID	
Rm Loranthi	Sang Ji Sheng 桑寄生	bitter neutral	"	
Carapax Amydae	Bie Jia 鱉甲	salty neutral	"	yin Def.—raw hardenings—use with vinegar
Plastrum Testudinis	Gui Ban 龜板	salty sweet neutral	"	
Sm Sesame	Hu Ma 胡麻	sweet neutral	LU, SP LIV, KID	
Mel (honey)	Feng Mi 蜂蜜	"	LU, SP LI	

1.Tonify LIV/KID 2.Brighten eyes	1.LIV/KID Deficiency 2.LIV/KID Def.-visual disturbances	9-15
1.Dispel Wind & Damp 2.Tonify KID/LIV 3.Nourish Body Fluids 4.Stabalize fetus	1.Def. Bi syndrome 2.hypermotility of fetus	9-18
1.Subdue Yang 2.Soften Hardenings	1.KID Yin Deficiency 2.LIV Yang Rising 3.SP/LIV enlargement	9-30
1.Subdue Yang 2.Tonify KID 3.Strengthen bones	1.LIV Yang Rising 2.KID Yin Deficiency 3.weak bones	9-30
1.Tonify LIV/KID 2.Lubricate Intestines 3.Nourish Blood	1.LIV/KID Deficiency 2.constipation 3.Yin & Blood Def.	9-30

1.Strengthen LU, Stop Cough
2.Lubricate Intestines
3.Strengthen ST & SP
	1.dry/chronic cough,
	  sore throat
	2.dry stool, constip.-
	  of old age
	3.ulcer, chronic hepat-
	  itis
		15-30

CHAPTER 20

ASTRINGENT HERBS

DEFINITION: Herbs that have astringing, contracting, and consolidating properties are used in a wide variety of disorders characterized by abnormal discharging of body substances. They are classified under this category.

GENERALIZATION: Most of these herbs are <u>astringent</u> and sour. Each has different functions of stopping abnormal leakage of body substances due to weakness. When these leakage continues, one becomes further weakened because the energy "escapes" with the discharge. Examples of the herb actions include stop sweating, relieve diarrhea, reduce urination, stop bleeding, relieve coughing and stop leukorrhea and spermatorrhea.

Astringent herbs can be further classified into 3 subcategories based on the part of the body they act on. They are 1) Upper Jiao Astringents or Anhydrotic herbs 2) Middle Jiao Astringents or Antidiarrhetic herbs and 3) Lower Jiao Astringents or antiephidrotic herbs.

These herbs are mostly symptomatic in action, thus Tonic herbs must be combined to reinforce the Astringent action and take care of the underlying cause.

SYMPTOMATOLOGY: Deficiency of the body give rise to abnormal discharges such as spontaneous sweating, frequent urination, seminal emission, leukorrhea, and chronic diarrhea. When there is an abnormal leakage of Qi, one may see chronic recurring cough and prolapse of organs. Other symptoms of Deficiency will often accompany. (Please see Tonics chapter)

CAUTIONS AND CONTRAINDICATIONS: Astringent herbs have a "closing" effect on the body to prevent further body discharge, therefore, in cases of External conditions where the treatment is to promote body discharge to expel the Pathogen from the surface, these herbs would certainly not be suitable.

PHARMACOLOGICAL ACTIONS: Most of these herbs have strong antibiotic effects. Some directly stimulate the central nervous system and have vasodilation actions while others increase the resting time in the intestinal peristalsis and strengthen the sphincter muscles in the bladder and the rectum.

SECTION ONE

UPPER JIAO ASTRINGENTS/ANHYDROTIC HERBS

DEFINITION: Herbs that act on the Upper Jiao to stop abnormal perspiration are considered to be Anhydrotic herbs.

GENERALIZATION: The energy of these herbs are said to be able to travel beneath the skin at the Wei (Defense) level to properly regulate the closing of the pores in order to stop abnormal sweating due to Deficient conditions. Abnormal sweating such as spontaneous sweat and night sweat have causes like Qi Deficiency, Yang Collapse, Yin Deficiency, Heart Fire and Phlegm Retention. Appropriate herbs must be combined to strengthen the Deficiencies. Other conditions such as Heart Fire and Phlegm Retention, one has to merely Clear the Fire and Resolve the Phlegm for the condition to recover.

SYMPTOMATOLOGY: Deficiency of the Upper Jiao (mainly the Lungs) may manifest as leakage of fluid or Qi as in spontaneous sweating and night sweat. In severe cases it can lead to Collapse of Yang such as in shock. In that instance, Herbs to restore the Yang must be administered.

CAUTIONS AND CONTRAINDICATIONS: Refrain from use in patients with External conditions.

SECTION TWO

MIDDLE JIAO ASTRINGENTS/ANTIDIARRHETIC HERBS

DEFINITION: Herbs that Astringe the Intestines to stop diarrhea are called Antidiarrhetic herbs.

GENERALIZATION: These herbs act to stop diarrhea by Astringing the Spleen and the Intestines. Diarrhea is often a symptom of Middle Jiao disharmony, in this case, it is the result of a Deficient Spleen. Sometimes Kidney Deficiency can accompany Spleen Deficient Diarrhea, therefore, proper Kidney Tonics along with Spleen Tonic herbs should also be administered. Some of the herbs have additional function of stopping bleeding and are most appropriate in chronic diarrhea with blood in the stools.

SYMPTOMATOLOGY: Chronic diarrhea sometimes daily at dawn, pale face, cold and heavy limbs, edema, prolapse of rectum or uterus, lower back and knee pain and weakness, lack of appetite, etc.

CAUTIONS AND CONTRAINDICATIONS: Do not use Antidiarrhetic herbs for diarrhea caused by Damp and Heat Factors.

156

SECTION THREE

LOWER JIAO ASTRINGENTS/ANTIEPHIDROTIC HERBS

DEFINITION: Herbs that reduce frequent urination, relieve leukorrhea and stop spermatorrhea by way of Astringing the Lower Jiao fall into this category.

GENERALIZATION: These herbs are mostly sweet and astringent in nature. They act on the Lower Jiao, mainly the Kidneys, to "hold-in" the essence and to prevent leakage of energy. Some have additional actions such as stopping cough due to inability of the Kidneys to Grasp the Qi from the Lungs, and arresting diarrhea that is a result of Spleen and Kidney weakness.

SYMPTOMATOLOGY: Frequent urination, bed wetting, premature ejaculation, seminal emission, chronic leukorrhea, pain and weakness in lower back and knees, ringing in the ear, blurry vision, infertility, diarrhea at dawn, chronic cough, etc.

CAUTIONS AND CONTRAINDICATIONS: Refrain from use in any Damp and Heat conditions.

CATEGORY: UPPER JAIO ASTRINGENT/ANHYDROTICS				
pharmaceutical name	pin-yin	taste & energy	meridians	comments
Fr Tritici	Fu Xiao Mai 浮小麥	sweet cool	HT	
Rx Ephedrae	Ma Huang Gen 麻黄根	sweet neutral	LU, HT	contra. external conditions

CATEGORY: MIDDLE JIAO ASTRINGENT/ANTIDIARRHETICS				
pharmaceutical name	pin-yin	taste & energy	meridian	comments
Galla Chinensis	Wu Bei Zi 五倍子	sour astrng cold	LU, LI KID	powder/pill form
Sm Myristicae	Rou Dou Kou 肉豆蔻	pungent warm	SP, ST LI	
Halloysitum Rubrum	Chi Shi Zhi 赤石脂	sweet astrng warm	"	contra. with Cx Cinnamomi contra. Damp Heat-diarrhea
Pericarpium Granati	Shi Liu Pi 石榴皮	sour astring warm	LI	
Fr Chebulae	He Zi 訶子	bitter sour astring neutral	LU, LI	

MAJOR ACTIONS: **ASTRINGE UPPER JIAO, STOP ABNORMAL PERSPIRATION**		
secondary actions	symptoms/conditions	dose (g)
1.Anti-hidrotic	1.spontaneous sweat, night sweat	9-30
1.Anti-hidrotic	1.spontaneous sweat, night sweat	3-9

MAJOR ACTIONS: **ASTRINGE MIDDLE JIAO, STOP DIARRHEA**		
1.Anti-hidrotic, Anti-diarrhetic 2.Stop bleeding	1.chronic diarrhea, spont./night sweat 2.LU Heat cough-Def.-with blood 3.bloody stool,urorrhea 4.ext-burns,hemorrhoids mouth ulcer, bleeding	.5-1.5
1.Anti-diarrhetic 2.Stop bleeding 3.Aid wound healing	1.chronic diarrhea 2.menorrhagia, leukor-rhea, bloody stool	6-24
1.Anti-diarrhetic 2.Warm Middle Jiao 3.Invigorate Qi	1.chronic diarrhea 2.Def. Cold of Middle Jiao-abd./epig. pain	3-9
1.Anti-diarrhetic 2.Anti-helminthic	1.chronic diarrhea 2.intestinal worms	3-5
1.Anti-diarrhetic 2.Clear Heat, Dry Damp	1.diarrhea, chronic dysentery,bloody stool, hemorrhoids 2.leukor.,menorrhagia	3-9

Cx Ailanthi 椿皮	Chun Pi	bitter astrng cold	LIV, LI	
Fr Mume 烏梅	Wu Mei	sour astring neutral	LIV, SP LU, LI	
Fr Papaveris 罌粟殼	Xing Su Ke	astring neutral toxic	LU, KI LI	contra. early stage diarrhea/cough or prolonged use

<table>
<tr><td colspan="5" align="center">CATEGORY: LOWER JIAO ASTRINGENT/ANTIEPHIDROTICS</td></tr>
<tr><th>pharmaceutical name</th><th>pin-yin</th><th>taste & energy</th><th>meridian</th><th>comments</th></tr>
<tr><td>Fr Schisandrae 五味子</td><td>Wu Wei Zi</td><td>sweet sour warm</td><td>KID, LU HT</td><td></td></tr>
<tr><td>Fr Corni 山茱萸</td><td>Shan Zhu Yu</td><td>sweet sour warm</td><td>LIV, KID</td><td></td></tr>
<tr><td>Fr Rubi 覆盆子</td><td>Fu Pen Zi</td><td>sweet sour sl.warm</td><td>"</td><td></td></tr>
<tr><td>Os Sepiae 海螵蛸</td><td>Hai Piao Xiao</td><td>salty sl.warm</td><td>LIV, KID ST</td><td>contra. with Rx Aconiti prolonged use may cause constipation</td></tr>
</table>

1.Anti-diarrhetic 2.Consolidate LU 3.Benefit throat	1.chronic diarrhea 2.chronic LU Def.-cough & loss of voice	3-9
1.Anti-diarrhetic 2.Consolidate LU 3.Nourish Body Fluids 4.Anti-helminthic	1.chronic diarrhea 2.chronic cough 3.Def. Heat-diabetes 4.intestinal worms-abd. pain/vomiting	3-9
1.Anti-diarrhetic 2.Consolidate LU 3.Stop pain	1.chronic diarrhea 2.chronic LU Def.-cough 3.epig. & abd. pain	3-9

MAJOR ACTIONS: **ASTRINGE LOWER JIAO, RETAIN THE ESSENCE**

1.Anti-ephidrotic, Anti-hidrotic
   Anti-diarrhetic
2.Tonify KID & HT
3.Tonify Qi, Nourish Body Fluids
	1.nocturnal emission,
	   chronic cough, sweat-
	   ing, chronic diarrhea
	2.insomnia
	3.Qi/Body Fluid Def.
		3-9

1.Anti-hidrotic
2.Anti-ephidrotic
3.Tonify KID & LIV
	1.spontaneous sweat,
	   night sweat
	2.nocturnal emission,
	   polyuria, enuresis
	3.impotence, back pain
		6-12

1.Anti-ephidrotic
2.Tonify KID & LIV
3.Brighten eyes
	1.nocturnal emission,
	   polyuria, enuresis
	2.KID & LIV Def.-blurry
	   vision
		9-15

1.Anti-ephidrotic
2.Stop bleeding
3.Soften Hardinings, Relieve
   Goitre
4.Aids wound healing
5.Neutralize ST acidity
	1.leukorrhea, seminal
	   emission
	2.blood in urine,stools
	   & vomit
	3.goitre, abscess
	4.ST hyperacidity,ulcer
		6-12

Sm Ginkgo	Bai Guo 白果	sweet bitter neutral astring toxic	LU	contra. cough with thick, tenacious phlegm Do not use raw — toxicity
Fr Rosae Laevigatae	Jin Ying Zi 金櫻子	sweet astring neutral	KID, UB LI	
Sm Nelumbinis	Lian Zi 蓮子	"	KID, SP HT	
Sm Eurayles	Qian Shi 芡實	"	SP, KID	

1.Anti-ephidrotic 2.Consolidates LU	1.leukorrhea, chyluria 2.chronic cough, asthma	6-9
1.Anti-ephidrotic 2.Anti-diarrhetic	1.nocturnal emimssion, polyuria, enuresis 2.chronic diarrhea 3.leukorrhea	4-9

1.Anti-ephidrotic
2.Anti-diarrhetic
	1.spont. sem. emission
	  leukorrhea, urorrhea
	  freq. micturition
	2.chronic diarrhea
		9-15

1.Anti-ephidrotic
2.Anti-diarrhetic
3.Nourish HT, Calm Spirit
	1.nocturnal emmission,
	  polyuria, enuresis,
	  leukorrhea
	2.chronic diarrhea
	3.insomnia, palpatation
		9-18

CHAPTER 21

TOPICAL HERBS

DEFINITION: Herbs that are used mainly for external purposes are called Topical herbs.

GENERALIZATION: The utilization of these topicals are a part of methods of External treatment. Each herb has a primary function such as Reduce swelling and detoxify, Resolve abscess and draw-out the poison, Invigorate blood and relieve pain, stop bleeding and relieve itching. They are applied in various ways like making the herbs into a paste, wash, powder, liquid drops, liniment and so forth and apply them to the affected areas of the body. There are herbs from other categories that can be used also for external purposes such as herbs that Clear Heat and Detoxify.

SYMPTOMATOLOGY: Topical herbs are used in many conditions of skin lesions and external cuts and burns. Examples of skin lesions include boils, carbuncles, rash, ulcers, warts, scabies, tinea, eczema, fungus infestation, ring worms, snake bites, infections of sensory organs, etc.

CAUTIONS AND CONTRAINDICATIONS: Many Topical herbs are <u>toxic</u>. Some can be taken internally, thus, one must use them with caution and closely regulate the amount and duration of usage so as not to cause side effects.

PHARMACOLOGICAL ACTIONS: Most herbs have been found to have antifungal, antibiotic, antimicrobial effects while some have local anesthetic, anti-inflammatory and antitumor effects in addition.

CATEGORY: TOPICAL HERBS				
pharmaceutical name	pin-yin	taste & energy	meridians	comments
Alumen	Ming Fan 明礬	sour astring cold	LU, SP LIV	use powdered
Fr Cnidii	She Chuang Zi 蛇床子	pungent bitter warm	KID	
Sulphur	Liu Huang 硫黄	sweet warm sl.tox	SP, KID	
Caulis Cinnamomi (Camphora)	Zhang Nao 樟腦	pungent hot toxic	HT	contra pregnant or Deficient overdose can kill
Secretio Bufonis	Chan Su 蟾酥	pungent warm toxic	"	contra pregnant avoid eyes
Sm Strychni	Ma Qian Zi 馬錢子	bitter cold toxic	ST, LIV	contra pregnant large dose may cause convulsion
Catechu seu Gambier	Er Cha 兒茶	bitter astring neutral		powder/pill form
Borax	Peng Sha 硼砂	sweet salty cool	LU, ST	contra. pregnant

MAJOR ACTIONS: DETOXIFY, RESOLVE SKIN LESIONS		
secondary actions	symptoms/conditions	dose (g)
1.ext-Astringe wounds 2.ext-Stop itching 3.int-Resolve Phlegm 4.int-Antidiarrhetic 5.int-Detoxify	1.chronic open wounds 2.skin lesions 3.epilepsy 4.chronic diarrhea 5.hepatitis, jaundice	1.5-3
1.ext-Antihelminthic 2.ext-Stop itching 3.int-Tonify KID Yang	1.trichomonis 2.itching 3.impotence, inertility	6-15
1.ext-Antihelminthic, Detoxify 2.int-Strengthen Ming Men Fire	1.skin lesions, itching 2.KID Yang Def.	1-3
1.ext-Dispel Damp 2.ext-Antihelminthic 3.ext-Reduce swelling, Stop pain 4.ext/int-Clear Orifices	1.tinea, impetigo 2.traumas 3.Turbidity obstructing Orifices	.03-.06
1.ext-Detoxify 2.ext-Stop pain 3.int-Clear Orifices	1.skin lesions 2.toothache, anaesthesia 3.Turbidity obtructing Orifices	.015-.3
1.ext/int-Detoxify 2.ext/int-Disperse Hardenings 3.ext/int-Invigorate Collaterals 4.ext/int-Stop pain	1.gastric, hepatic, lung, breast carcinoma 2.Bi syndrome	.3-.6
1.ext-Astringe wounds 2.ext/int-Astringent hemostatic	1.suppurative skin les. 2.internal bleeding	1-3

1.ext-Clear Heat, Detoxify
2.int-Clear Heat, Resolve Phlegm
	1.ulcerated tongue,
	   conjunctivitis,
	   laryngo-pharyngitis
	2.LU Heat cough
		3-6

CHAPTER 22

EMETIC HERBS

DEFINITION: An herb that induces vomiting is considered an Emetic herb.

GENERALIZATION: Emetic herbs have the major action of artificially inducing vomiting for the purpose of expelling unwanted substance from the body. They tend to be toxic and may cause drastic reactions to the body, therefore, exercise extreme caution when administering Emetic herbs.

According to the ancient classics, it is said that when the pathogen is lodged high up in the trunk, expel it through vomiting. Vomiting is one of the three main methods of treatment emphasized by the "Zhang Zi He School" in Traditional Chinese Medicine during the Yuan Dynasty. The other two methods are sweating and purging. In modern times, unless a condition such as poisoning which calls for immediately expelling through regurgitation, the method of vomiting is seldom used anymore because of its drastic results and possible side effects. However, Emetic herbs can still be used to beneficial effects when used correctly. Conditions indicated for Emetic herbs are food or drug poisoning, food retention, and copious phlegm as in cases of Damp-Phlegm or epilepsy and seizures.

If after taking the herbs, the vomiting becomes unbearable, to stop vomiting, one merely has to drink some cold water to neutralize the effects.

SYMPTOMATOLOGY: Emetic herbs can be used in conditions of poisoning or overdose through food or drugs whereby an effort is made to excrete the substances quickly before it becomes assimilated into the body. This is especially useful in cases of children ingesting toxic materials such as lead paint and household liquids, to mention a few. If one can get the child to vomit the substance out in time, one can save the child from great harm. In cases of poisoning like the ones mentioned above, one is usually relatively symptom-free until the substances become absorbed into the system. By that time, it is usually too late to administer Emetic herbs. However, when one encounters food retention in the stomach or esophagus, common symptoms are fullness and distention in the chest and stomach area, sometimes pain may be present with acid regurgitation. In these cases, one may chose to use Emetic herbs to relieve the obstruction from the gastro-intestinal track by getting rid of the stagnant food.

Another area of application is in cases where there are presence of copious phlegm accumulated in the lungs that is causing trouble with breathing, pressure and fullness in the chest. In this case, emetic herbs would be effective in expectorate the excess phlegm from the lungs.

Emetic herbs can also be utilized in epilepsy and seizure conditions that are accompanied by foaming at the mouth, and stridor (rattling noise in the throat from phlegm obstruction). These conditions in Chinese Medicine are most likely due to Wind and Phlegm masking and clogging the Orifice (Heart and sensory), thus, expelling the Phlegm would be an essential part of an effective treatment.

CONTRAINDICATIONS: Because of its toxicity and drastic actions, Emetic herbs are not recommended for old and weak patients, people with hypertension, pregnant women, postpartum and bleeding persons.

	CATEGORY: EMETIC HERBS

pharmaceutical name	pin-yin	taste & energy	meridians	comments
Rx Veratri	Li Lu 藜蘆	pungent cold toxic	SP, ST LU	contra. pregnant contra. with
Calyx Melonis	Gua Di 瓜蒂	bitter cold toxic	SP, ST GB	use in powder form

MAJOR ACTIONS: **PROMOTE EMESIS**		
secondary actions	symptoms/conditions	dose (g)
1. Resolve Phlegm 2. Anti-helminthic	1. seizures, epilepsy, stroke due to Wind-Phlegm	.3-1
1. Relieve jaundice	1. Phlegm Damp accumulation, ext-jaundice 2. food retention	.3-1

HERB SAMPLES

SCALE: Each unit represents one inch

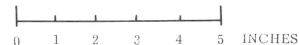

0   1   2   3   4   5   INCHES

* ALL HERB SAMPLES ARE PICTURED TO SCALE

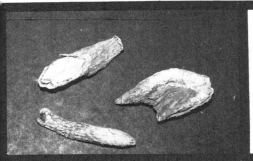

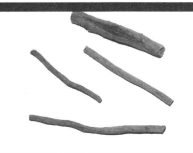

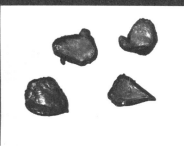

Cx Acanthopanacis

WU JIA PI   五加皮

Rx Achyranthis Bid.

NIU XI   牛膝

Rx Aconiti Carm. Prep.

FU ZI   附子

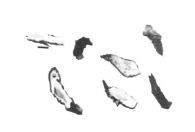

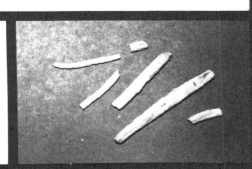

Rx Aconiti Coreani

BAI FU ZI   白附子

Rz Acori Graminei

SHI CHANG PU

石菖蒲

Rx Adenophorae

NAN SHA SHEN

南沙参

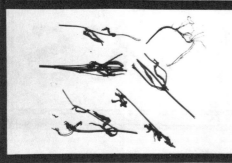

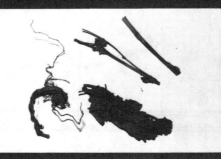

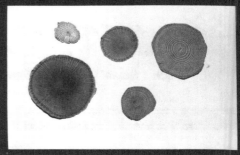

Hb Agastachis (Pogostemi)

HUO XIANG 藿香

Hb Agrimoniae

XIAN HE CAO

仙鶴草

Caulis Akebiae

MU TONG 木通

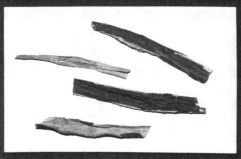

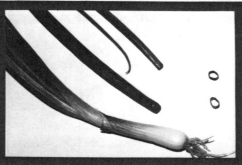

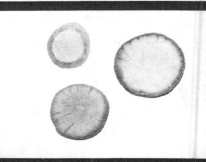

Cx Albizzii

HE HUAN PI 合欢皮

Bulbus Allium

CONG BAI 葱白

Rz Alismatis

ZE XIE 澤泻

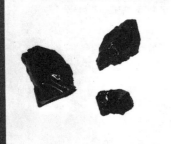

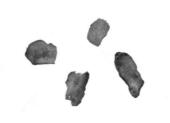

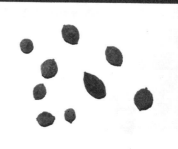

Hb Aloes

LU HUI 芦荟

Rz Alpiniae

GAO LIANG JIANG

高良姜

Fr Alpiniae Oxyphyllae

YI ZHI REN 益智仁

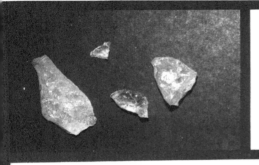

Alumen

BAI FAN　白矾

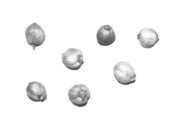

Fr seu Sm Amomi

SHA REN　砂仁

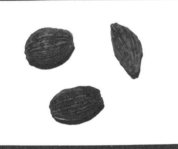

Fr Amomi Cardamomi

DOU KOU　豆蔻

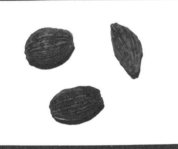

Fr Amomi Tsaokou

CAO GUO　草果

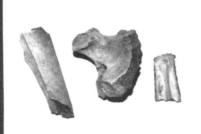

Carapax Amydae

BIE JIA　鳖甲

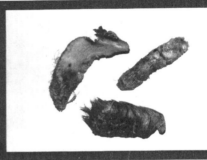

Rz Anamarrhenae

ZHI MU　知母

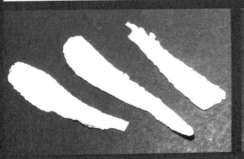

Rx Angelicae Dahuricae

BAI ZHI　白芷

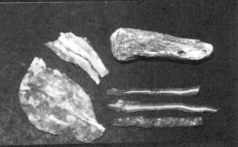

Rx Angelicae Sinensis

DANG GUI　当归

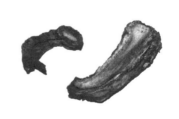

Rx Angelicae Tuhuo

DU HUO　独活

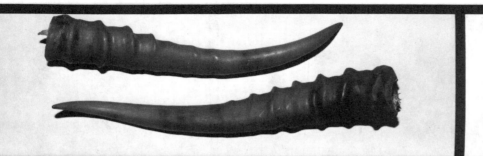

Cornu Antelopis

LING YANG JIAO 羚羊角

Fr Arctii

NIU BANG ZI 牛蒡子

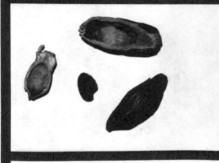

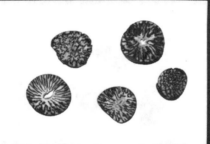

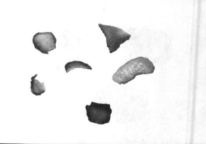

Pericarpium Arecae

DA FU PI 大腹皮

Sm Arecae

BING LANG 槟榔

Rz Arisaematis

TIAN NAN XING

天南星

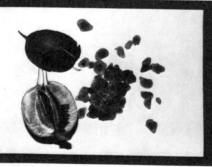

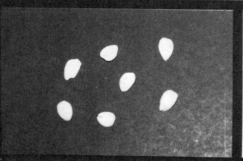

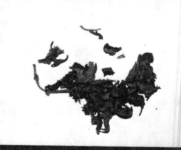

Fr Aristolochiae

MA DOU LING

馬兜鈴

Sm Armeniacae

XING REN 杏仁

Fm Artemesiae Argyii

AI YE 艾叶

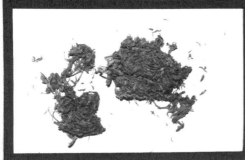

Hb Artemesiae Capillaris

YIN CHEN 茵陳

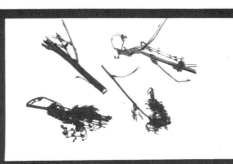

Hb Artemesiae Chinghao

CHING HAO 青蒿

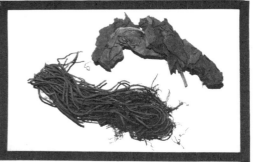

Hb Asari cum Radice

XI XIN 細辛

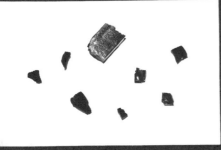

Gelatinum Asini (Nigra)

E JIAO 阿胶

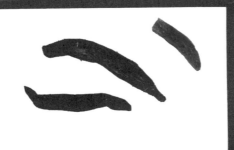

Rx Asparagi

TIAN MEN DONG 天門冬

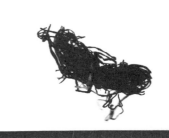

Rx Asteris

ZI WAN 紫菀

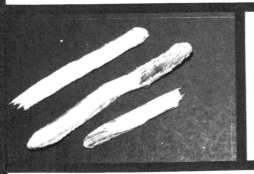

Rx Astragali

HUANG QI 黄芪

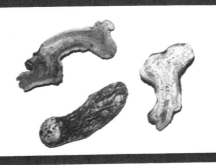

Rz Atractylodes Alba

BAI ZHU 白术

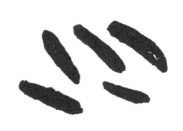

Fr Aurantii

ZHI KE 枳壳

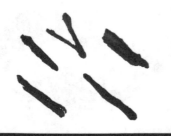

Fr Aurantii Immaturis

ZHI SHI (Ponciri) 枳实

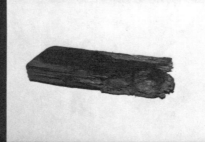

Lignum Aquilariae

CHEN XIANG 沉香

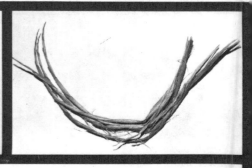

Bambosae en Taenia

ZHU RU 竹茹

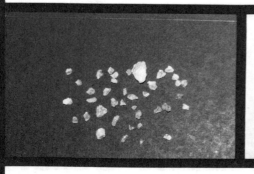

Benzoinum

AN XI XIANG 安息香

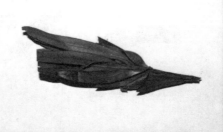

Caucumen Biotae

CE BAI YE 侧柏叶

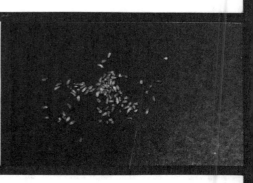

Sm Biotae

BAI ZI REN 柏子仁

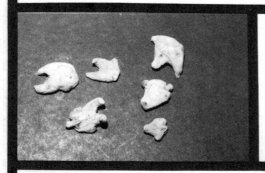

Rz Bletillae

BAI JI 白芨

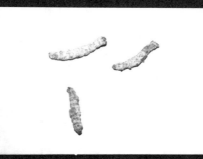

Bombyx Batriticatus

JIANG CAN 僵蚕

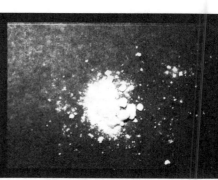

Borax

MING FAN 明矾

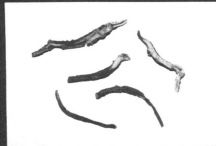
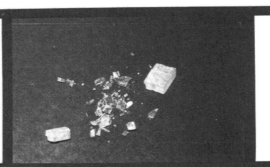
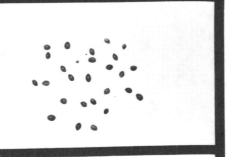

Rx Bupleuri

CHAI HU　柴胡

Calcitum

HAN SHUI SHI
寒水石

Sm Cannabis

HUO MA REN
火麻仁

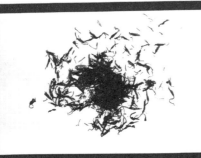
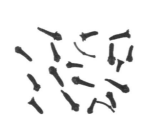
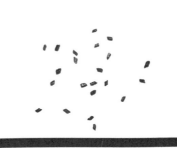

Fl Carthami

HONG HUA　紅花

Fl Caryophyllae

DING XIANG　丁香

Sm Cassiae Torrae

JUE MING ZI
决明子

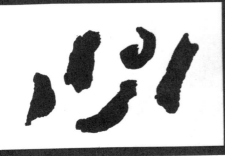
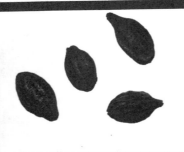
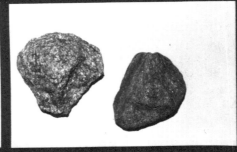

Fr Chaenomelis

MU GUA　木瓜

Fr Chebulae

HE ZI　訶子

Chloriti (Lapis)

MENG SHI　礞石

179

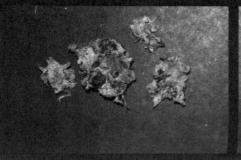
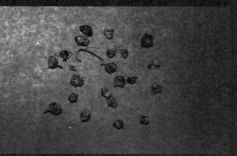
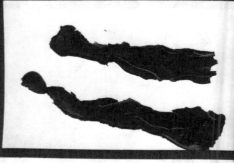

Fl Chrysanthemi

JU HUA　菊花

Fl Chrysanthemi Indicum

YE JU HUA　野菊花

Rz Cibotii

GOU JI　狗脊

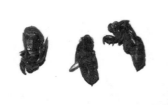
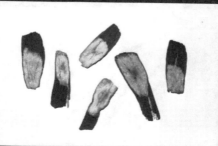
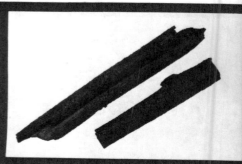

Periostracum Cicadae

CHAN TUI　蝉蜕

Rz Cimicifugae

SHENG MA　升麻

Cx Cinnamomi

GUI PI　肉桂

(ROU GUI)

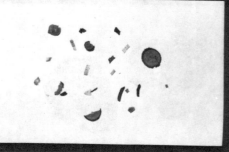
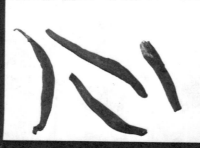
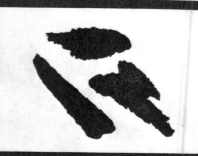

Rm Cinnamomi

GUI ZHI　桂枝

Hb Cirsii Japonici

DA JI　大蓟

Hb et Rx Cistanchis

ROU CONG RONG

肉苁蓉

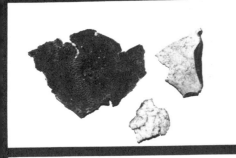

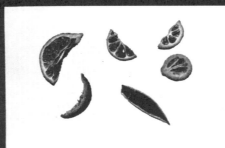

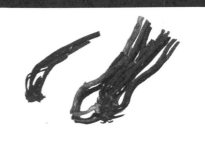

Peric. Citri Retic.

CHEN PI 陳皮

Peric. Citri Retic. Verde

QING PI 青皮

Rx Clematidis

WEI LING XIAN 威灵仙

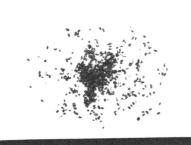

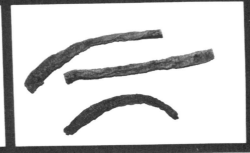

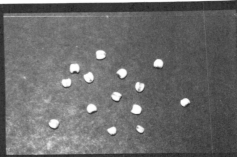

Fr Cnidii

SHE CHUANG ZI 蛇床子

Rx Codonopsis

DANG SHENG 党参

Sm Coicis

YI YI REN 薏苡仁

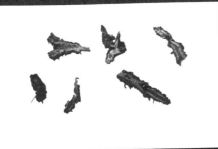

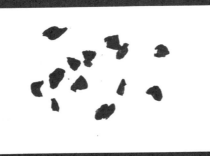

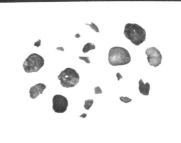

Rz Coptidis

HUANG LIAN 黄連

Fr Corni

SHAN ZHU YU 山茱萸

Rz Corydalis

YAN HU SUO 延胡索

181

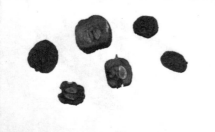

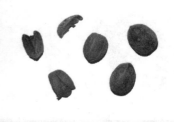

Fr Crataegi

SHAN ZHA　山楂

Crinis Carbonisatus

XUE YU TAN　血余炭

Sm Crotonis

BA DOU　巴豆

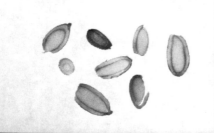

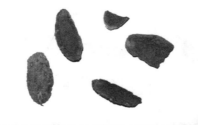

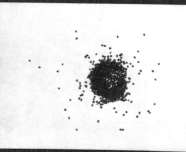

Rx Curcumae

YU JIN　郁金

Rz Curcumae Longae

JIANG HUANG　姜黄

Sm Cuscutae

TU SI ZI　菟絲子

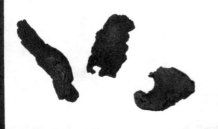

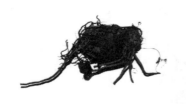

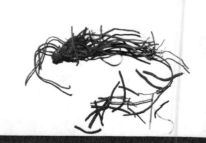

Hb Cynamori

SUO YANG　鎖陽

Rx Cynanchi Atrati

BAI WEI　白薇

Rx Cynanchi Stautoni

BAI QIAN　白前

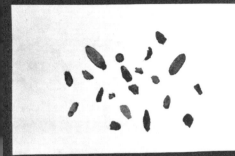

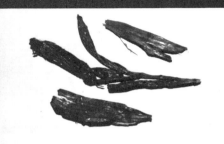

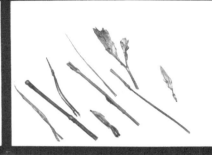

Rz Cyperi

XIANG FU 香附

Hb Dendrobi

SHI HU 石斛

Hb Dianthi

QU MAI 瞿麦

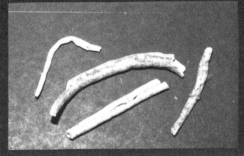

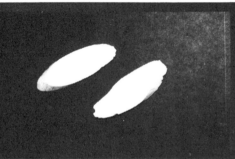

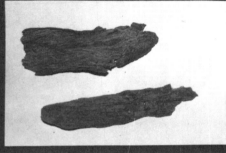

Cx Dictamni Radicis

BAI XIAN PI

白蘚皮

Rx Dioscorea

SHAN YAO 山药

Rx Dipsaci

XU DUAN 續斷

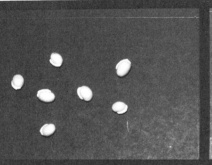

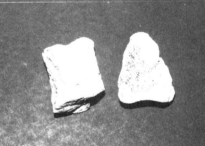

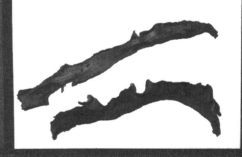

Sm Dolichoris

BAI BIAN DOU

白扁豆

Os Draconis

LONG GU 龍骨

Rz Drynariae

GU SUI BU 骨碎補

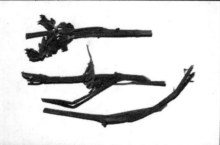

Hb Elsholtziae

XIANG RU 香薷

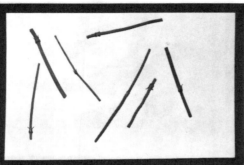

Hb Ephedrae

MA HUANG 麻黄

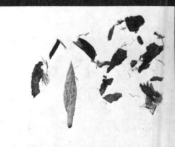

Rx Ephedrae

MA HUANG GEN 麻黄根

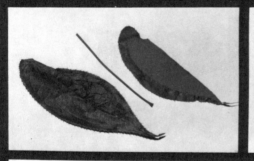

Hb Epimedii

YIN YANG HUO 淫羊藿

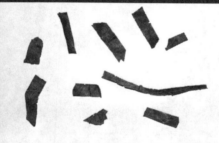

Fm Eriobotryae

PI PA YE 枇杷叶

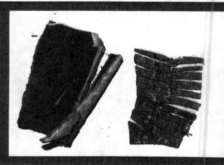

Cx Eucommiae

DU ZHONG 杜仲

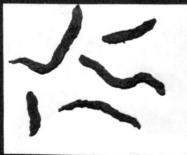

Rz Euphorbiae Pekinensis

DA JI 大戟

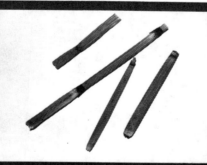

Hb Equiseti

MU ZEI 木贼

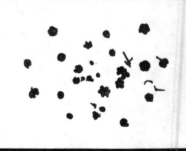

Fr Evodiae

WU ZHU YU 吴茱萸

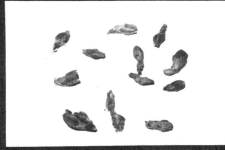

Fl Farfarae

KUAN DONG HUA

款冬花

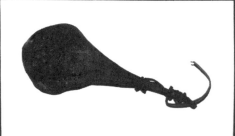

Fel Ursi

XIONG DAN　熊胆

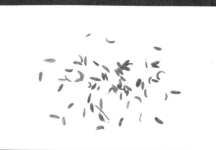

Fr Foeneculi

HUI XIANG

小茴香

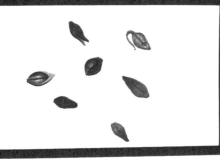

Fr Forsythiae

LIAN QIAO　連翹

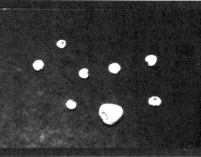

Bulbus Fritillariae Cir.

CHUAN BEI MU

川貝母

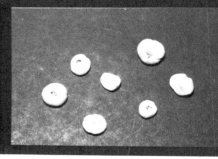

Bulbus Fritillariae Thunb.

ZHE BEI MU

浙貝母

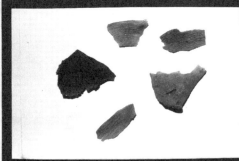

**Gallus Domesticus (Endo-
thelium Corneum Gigeriae
Galli) JI NEI JING**

鸡内金

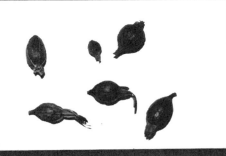

Fr Gardeniae

ZHI ZI　栀子

Rz Gastrodiae

TIAN MA　天麻

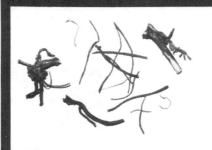
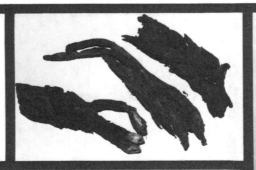
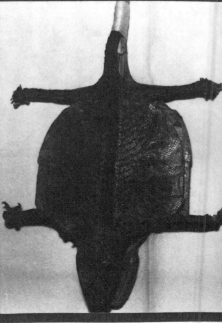

Rx Gentianae

LONG DAN CAO

龍胆草

Rx Gentianae Macro.

QIN JIAO 秦艽

Gecko

GE JIE 蛤蚧

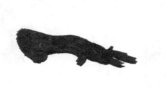
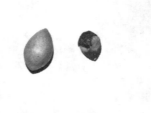

Rx Ginseng

REN SHEN 人参

Sm Ginkgo

BAI GUO 白果

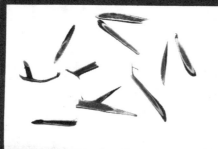
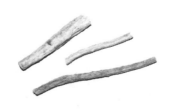
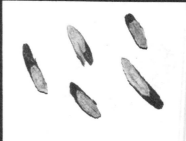

Spina Gleditsiae

ZAO JIAO CI

皂角刺

Rx Glehniae

SHA SHEN 沙参(北)

Rx Glycyrrhizae

GAN CAO 甘草

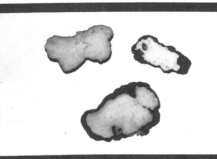
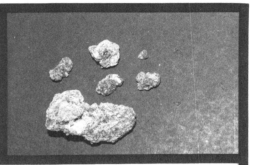

Pericarpium Granati

SHI LIU PI 石榴皮

Grifolia

ZHU LING 豬苓

Gummi Olibanum

RU XIANG 乳香

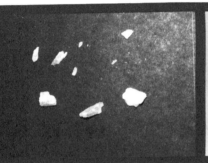
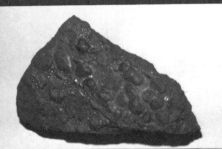
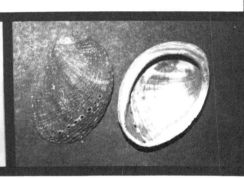

Gypsum Fibrosum

SHI GAO 石膏

Hematitum

DAI ZHE SHI 代赭石

Haliotidis

SHI JUE MING 石决明

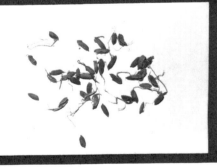
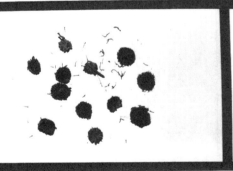
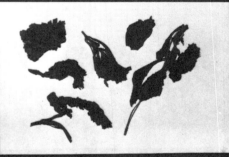

Fr Hordeum

MAI YA 麦芽

Fl Inulae

XUAN FU HUA 旋复花

Fm Isatidis

DA QING YE 大青叶

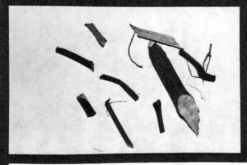
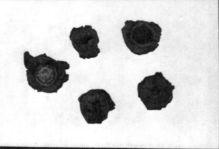
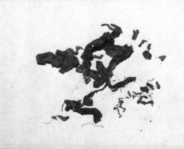

Rx Isatis	**Calyx Kaki**	**Hb Laminariae**
BAN LAN GEN	SHI DI 柿蒂	KUN BU 昆布
板藍根		

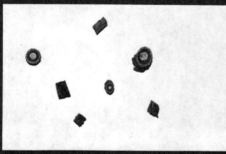
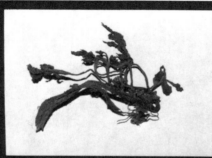
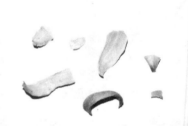

Hb Ledebourelliae (Siler)	**Hb Leonuri**	**Bulbus Lilii**
FANG FENG 防风	YI MU CAO 益母草	BAI HE 百合

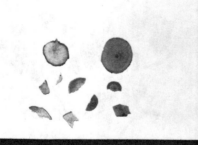
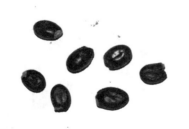
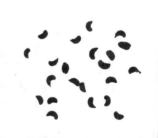

Rx Linderae	**Sm Litchi**	**Fr Ligustici Lucidi**
WU YAO 烏葯	LI ZHI 荔枝	NU ZHEN ZI
		女貞子

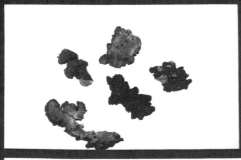

Rx et Rz Ligustici

GAO BEN 藁本

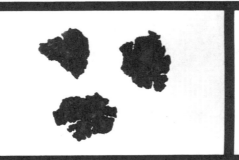

Rx Ligustici Wallichi

CHUAN XIONG 川芎

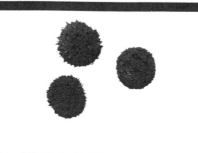

Liquidamber

LU LU TONG 路路通

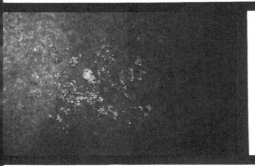

Stryax Liquidius

SU HE XIANG 蘇合香

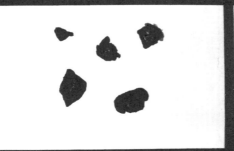

Arillus Longanae

LONG YAN ROU 龍眼肉

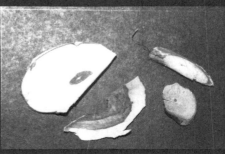

Caulis Lonicerae

REN DONG TENG 忍冬苍

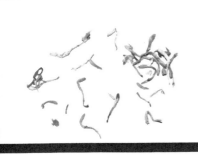

Fl Lonicerae

JIN YIN HUA 金銀花

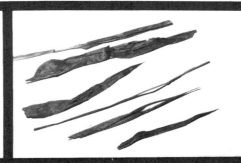

Hb Lophatheri

DAN ZHU YE 淡竹叶

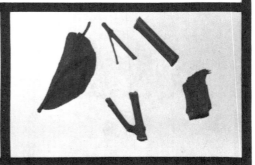

Rm Loranthi

SANG JI SHEN 桑寄生

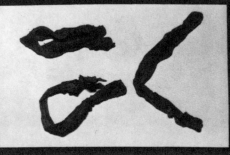
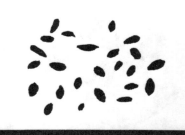

Lumbricus	**Cx Lycii Radicis**	**Fr Lycium**
DI LONG 地龍	DI GU PI 地骨皮	GOU QI ZI 枸杞子

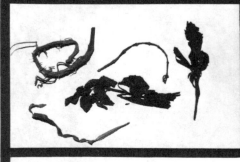
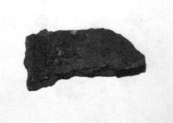
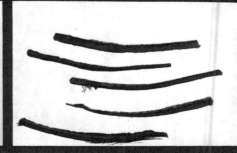

Hb Lycopi	**Magnetitum**	**Cx Magnoliae**
ZE LAN 澤蘭	CI SHI 磁石	HOU PO 厚朴

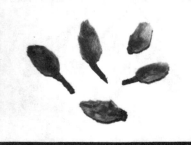
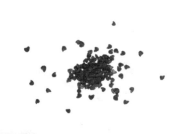
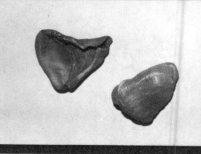

Fl Magnoliae Liliflorae	**Sm Malvae**	**Squama Manitis**
XIN YI 辛荑	DONG KUEI ZI 冬葵子	CHUAN SHAN JIA 穿山甲

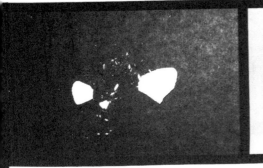

Margaritifera

(Choncha Margarita)

ZHEN ZHU MU 珍珠母

Massa Fermentata

SHEN QU 神袖

Medulla Junci

DENG XIN CAO 燈心草

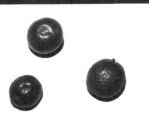
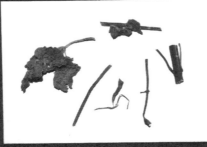
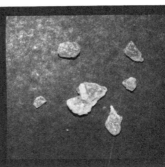

Fr Meliae Toosendan

CHUAN LIAN ZI

川棟子

Hb Menthae

BO HE 薄荷

Mirabilitum Depuratum

MANG XIAO 芒硝

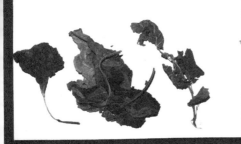
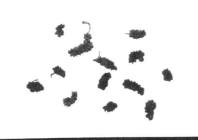
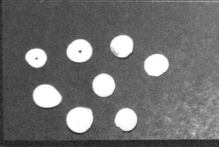

Fm Mori

SANG YE 桑叶

Fr Mori

SANG SHAN 桑椹

Rm Mori

SANG ZHI 桑枝

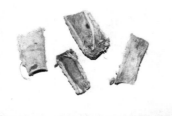

Cx Mori Radicis

SANG BAI PI

桑白皮

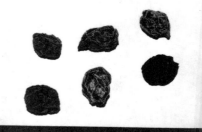

Rx Morindae

BA JI TIAN

巴戟天

Fr Mume

WU MEI 烏梅

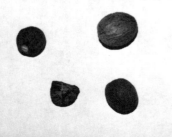

Sm Myristicae

ROU DOU KOU

肉豆蔻

Commiphora Myrrha

MO YAO 没葯

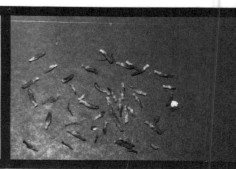

Plumula Nelumbinis

LIAN ZI XIN

蓮子芯

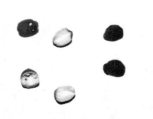

Sm Nelumbinis

LIAN ZI 蓮子

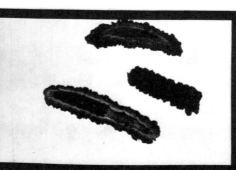

Rx et Rz Notopterygii

QIANG HUO 羌活

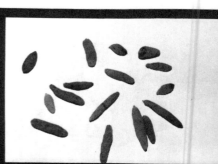

Rx Ophiopogonis

MAI MEN DONG

麦門冬

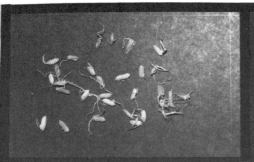

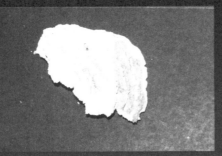

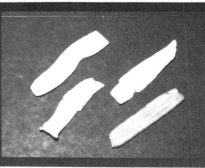

Fr Oryzae

GU YA 谷芽

Concha Ostrea

MU LI 牡蛎

Rx Paeoniae Alba

BAI SHAO

白芍

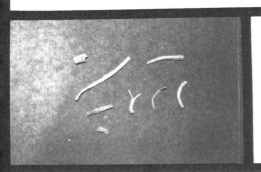

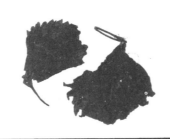

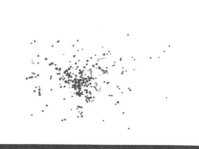
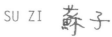

Rx Panacis Quinquefolii

XI YANG SHEN

西洋参

Fm Perillae

SU YE 蘇叶

Fr et Sm Perillae

SU ZI 蘇子

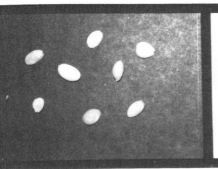

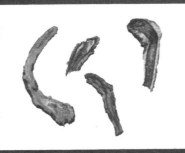

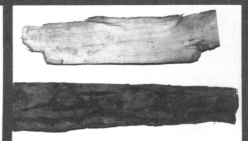

Sm Persicae

TAO REN 桃仁

Rx Peucedani

QIAN HU 前胡

Cx Phellodendri

HUANG BAI 黄柏

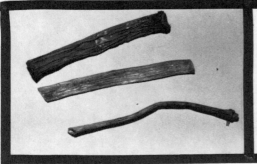

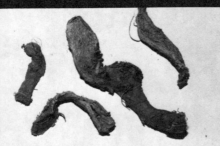

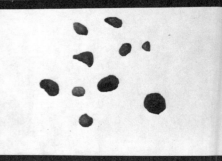

Rx Phragmites

LU GEN   芦根

Rx Phytolaccae

SHANG LU   离陆

Rz Pinelliae

BAN XIA

半夏

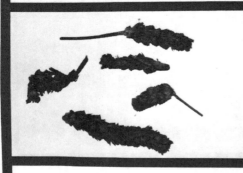

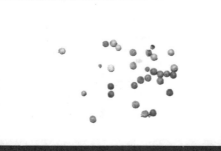

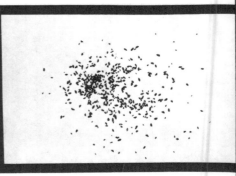

Spika Prunella

SHA KU CAO   夏枯草

Fr Piperi Nigri

HU JIAO   胡椒

Sm Plantaginis

CHE QIAN ZI

車前子

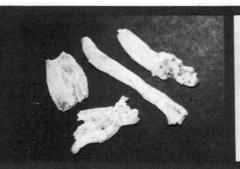

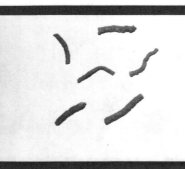

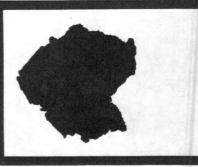

Rx Platycodi

JIE GENG   桔梗

Rx Polygala

YUAN ZHI   遠志.

Rx Polygonati

HUANG JING   黄精

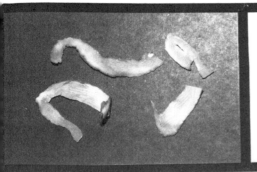
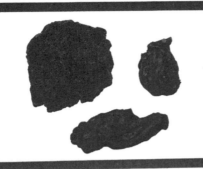
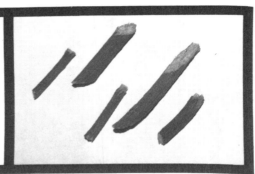

Rx Polygoni Officinalis

YU ZHU　　玉竹

Rx Polygoni Multiflori

HE SHOU WU　　何首烏

Caulis Polygoni Multiflori

YE JIAO TENG

夜交莧

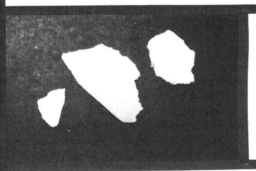
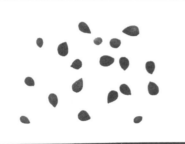
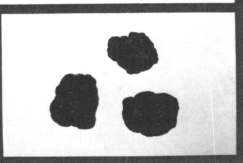

Poria Cocos

FU LING　　茯苓

Sm Pruni

YU LI REN　　郁李仁

Rx Pseudoginseng

SAN QI　　三七

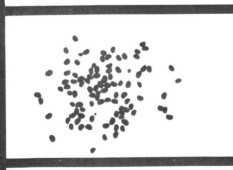
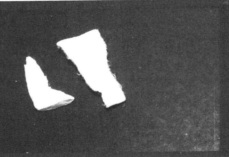
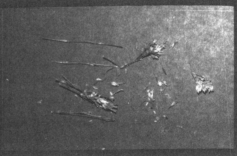

Fr Psoraleae

BU GU ZHI　　補骨脂

Rx Puerariae

GE GEN　　葛根

Rx Pulsatillae

BAI TOU WENG

白頭翁

195

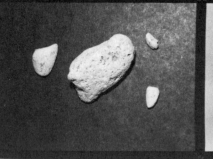
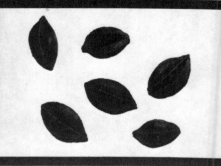
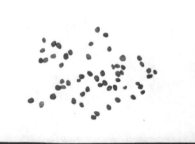

Pumice

HAI FU SHI 海浮石

Pyritum

ZI RAN TONG 自然銅

Fr Quisqualis

SHI JUN ZI 使君子

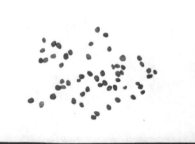
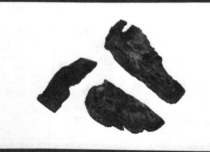

Sm Raphani

LAI FU ZI 萊菔子

Rz Rhei

DA HUANG 大黃

Rx Rehmanniae (cooked)

SHU DI HUANG 熟地黃

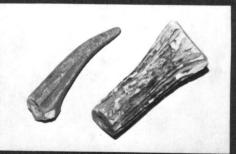
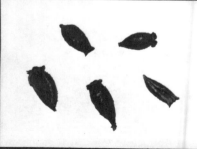

Rx Rehmanniae (raw)

SHENG DI HUANG 生地黃

Cornu Rhinoceri

XI JIAO 犀角

Fr Rosae Laevigatae

JIN YIN ZI 金櫻子

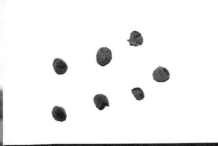

Fr Rubi

FU PEN ZI 覆盆子

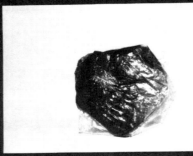

Saccharum Granorum

YI TANG 飴糖

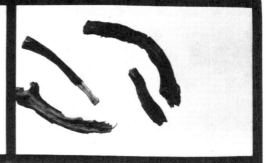

Rx Salviae Multiorrhizae

DAN SHEN 丹参

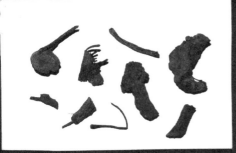

Rx Sanguisorbae

DI YU 地榆

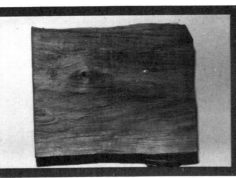

Lignum Santali

TAN XIANG 檀香

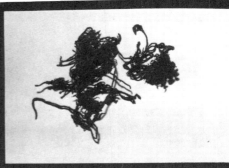

Sargassum

HAI ZAO 海藻

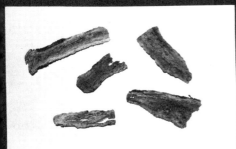

Rx Saussureae

MU XIANG 木香

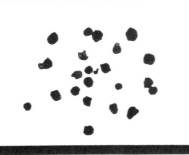

Fr Schizandrae

WU WEI ZI 五味子

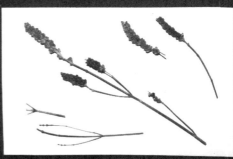

Hb Schizonepetae

JING JIE 荆芥

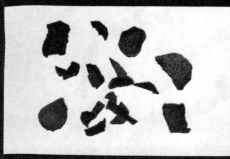

Rz Scirbii (Sparganii)

SAN LENG 三棱

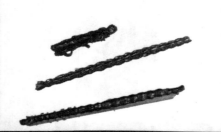

Scolopendrae

WU GONG 蜈蚣

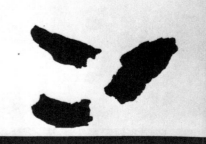

Rx Scrophulariae

XUAN SHEN 玄参

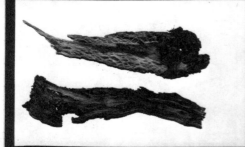

Rx Scutellariae

HUANG QIN 黄芩

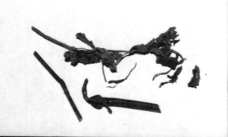

Hb Siegesbeckiae

XI XIAN 豨莶

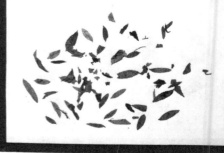

Fm Sennae

FAN XIE YE

番泻叶

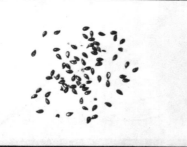

Sm Sesame

HU MA REN 火麻仁

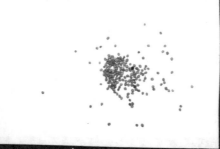

Sm Sinapis Alba

BAI JIE ZI

白芥子

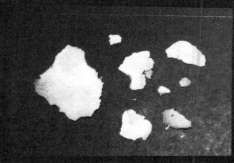

Rz Smilacis Glabrae

TU FU LING

土茯苓

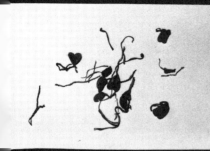

Sm Sojae Germinatum

DA DOU HUANG JUAN

大豆黄卷

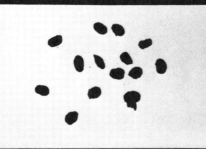

Sm Sojae Praeparatae

(DAN) DOU CHI

淡豆豉

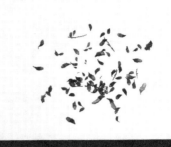

Fl Sophorae

HUAI HUA 槐花

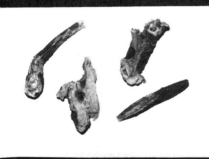

Rx Sophorae Flavesentis

KU SHEN 苦參

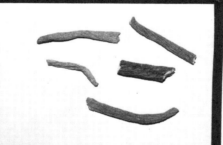

Rx Stellariae

YIN CHAI HU

銀柴胡

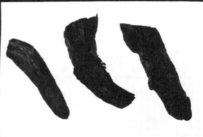

Rx Stemonae

BAI BU 百部

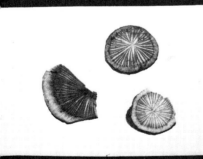

Rx Stephaniae

FANG JI 防己

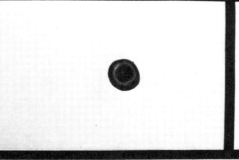

S Strychni

MA QIAN ZI 馬錢子

Sulphur

LIU HUANG 硫黄

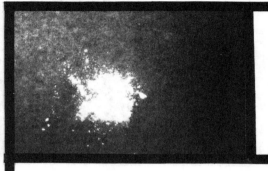

Talcum

HUA SHI 滑石

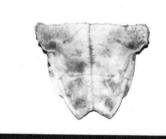

Plastrum Testudinis

GUI BAN 龟板

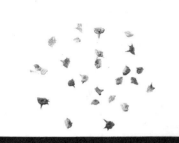

Fr Tribuli

BAI JI LI 白蒺藜

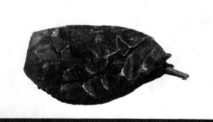

Fr Trichosanthis

(QUAN) GUA LOU 全瓜蒌

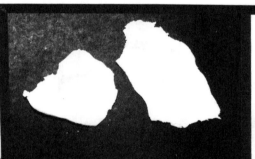

Rx Trichosanthis

TIAN HUA FEN 天花粉

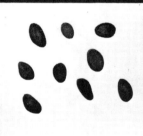

Sm Trichosanthis

GUA LOU REN 瓜蒌仁

Fr Tritici

FU XIAO MAI 浮小麦

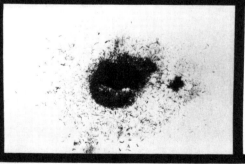

Pollen Typhae

PU HUANG 蒲黄

Rm Uncariae cum Uncis

GOU TENG 钩芎

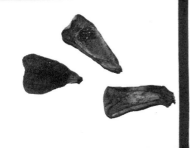

Sm Vacarriae

WANG BU LIU XING

王不留行

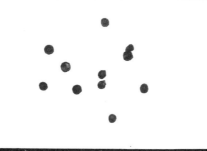

Fr Viticis

MAN JING ZI

蔓荆子

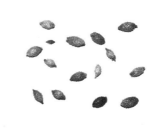

Fr Xanthii

CANG ER ZI

蒼耳子

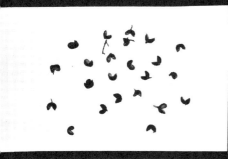

Fr Zanthoxyli

SHU JIAO 花椒

（蜀椒）

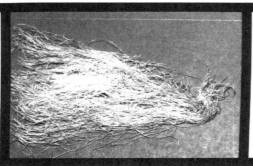

Stylus Zeae

YU MI XU 玉米鬚

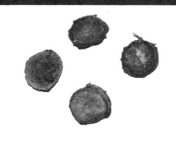

Rz Zedoariae

E ZHU 莪茂

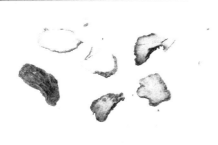

Rz Zingiberis

GAN JIANG 干姜

Fr Ziziphi Sativae

DA ZAO 大枣

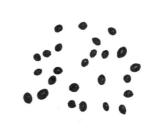

Sm Ziziphi Spinosae

SUAN ZAO REN

酸枣仁

201

BIBLIOGRAPHY

1. Beijing Collge of Traditional Chinese Medicine. <u>Discussion of Yellow Emperor's Classics of Internal Medicine (Nei Jing Jiang Yi)</u>. Hong Kong: Medicine and Hygiene Publisher, Hong Kong, 1975 (Chinese).

2. Chen Wei Hua, et.al. <u>Discussion of Herbal Combinations (Yao Dui Lun)</u>. An Hui, China: An Hui science and technical Press, 1983 (Chinese).

3. Chengdu College of Traditional Chinese Medicine, et.al. <u>Chinese Herbal Medicine (Zhong Yao Xue)</u>. Shanghai, China: Shanghai science and technical Press, 1978 (Chinese).

4. D. Bensky and A. Gamble. <u>Chinese Herbal Medicine: Materia Medica</u>. Seatle: Eastland Press, 1986 (English)

5. Gansu Provincial Academy of New Medicine, et.al. <u>Chinese Herbal Medicine (Zhong Yao Xue)</u>. Beijing, China: People's Hygiene Press, 1982 (Chinese).

6. Yeung, Him-Che. <u>Handbook of Chinese Herbs and Formulas</u>. 1983, (English).

7. Jiangsu College of New Medicine. <u>Encyclopedia of Materia Medica (Zhong Yao Da Ci Dian)</u>. Shanghai, China: People's Press, 1977 (Chinese).

8. Liu Bo Ji. <u>History of Chinese Medicine (Zhong Guo Yi Xue Shi)</u>. Taiwan: Hua Gang Press, 1974 (Chinese).

9. Nanjing College of Traditional Chinese Medicine. <u>Yellow Emperor's Classics of Internal Medicine: Simple Questions (Huang Di Nei Jing Su Wen Shi Yi)</u>. Shanghai, China: Shanghai science and technical Press, 1959 (Chinese).

10. Shanghai College of Traditional Chinese Medicine. <u>Classified Commonly Used Herbs and Formulas (Chung Yon Fang Yao Lei Bien)</u>. Shanghai, China: Shanghai science and technical Press, 1981 (Chinese).

APPENDIX A:

18 INCOMPATIBLE AND 19 ANTAGONISTIC HERBS

Traditionally, there have been observed that certain combination of usually two specific substances will render the substances useless. These substances are thus called the 19 Antagonisms because there are a total of 19 of them. In addition, some herbs have been found to react with side effects only when combined with another. These substances are said to be incompatible with one another. There are three sets with a total of 18 substances called the 18 Incompatibilities.

EIGHTEEN INCOMPATIBILITIES

Rx Glycyrrhizae (Gan Cao) is incompatible with:
      Rx Euphorbiae Kansui (Gan Sui)
      Rx Euphorbiae Seu Knoxiae (Da Ji)
      Fl Daphnes Genkwa (Yuan Hua)
      Hb Sargassii (Hai Zao)

Rx Aconiti (Wu Tou) is incompatible with:
      Bulbus Fritillariae (Bei Mu)
      Rz Pinelliae (Ban Xia)
      Fr Trichosanthis (Gua Lou)
      Rx Ampelopsis (Bai Lian)
      Rz Bletillae (Bai Ji)

Rz et Rx Veratri (Li Lu) is incompatible with:
      Rx Ginseng (Ren Shen)
      Rx Glehniae (Sha Shen)
      Rx Salviae Miltiorrhizae (Dan Shen)
      Rx Sophorae Flavescentis (Ku Shen)
      Hb Asari Cum Radicis (Xi Xin)
      Rx Paeoniae lactiflorae (Bai Shao)

NINETEEN ANTAGONISMS

    Sulphur (Liu Huang) antagonizes Sal Glauberis (Po Xiao)
    Hydrargyrum (Shui Yin) antagonizes Arsenicum (Pi Shuang)
    Rx Euphorbiae Fischerianae (Lang Du) antagonizes Lithargyrum (Mi Tuo Zhen)
    Sm Crotonis (Ba Dou) antagonizes Sm Pharbitidis (Qian Niu Zi)
    Nitrum (Ya Xiao) antagonizes Rz Sparganii (San Leng)
    Fl Caryophylli (Ding Xiang) antagonizes Rz Curcumae Longae (Yu Jin)
    Rx Aconiti (Wu Tou & Cao Wu) antagonizes Cornu Rhinoceri (Xi Jiao)
    Rx Ginseng (Ren Shen) antagonizes Excrementum Trogopterori (Wu Ling Zhi)
    Cx Cinnamomi (Rou Gui) antagonizes Halloysitum Rubrum (Chi Shi Zhi)

APPENDIX B: LIST OF CATEGORIES AND HERBS

DIAPHORETIC WARMING
Rx Angelicae Dihur.
Allium Fistulosum
Hb Elsholtziae
Fl Magnolia
Rz Zingiberis
 (fresh)
Fo Perillae
Hb Asari
Rx Ligustici
Hb Ledebourelia
Rm Cinnamomi
Fr Xanthii
Hb Ephedrae
Hb Schizonepeta
Rx Notopterygii

DIAPHORETIC COOLING
Hb Mentha
Peri Cicadae
Fl Chrysanthemi
Hb Equisetii
Fo Mori
Fr Viticis
Rx Puerariae
Rx Cimicifugae
Rx Bupleuri
Fr Arctii
Sm Sojae Preparata
Fl Chrysanthemi
 Indicum
Hb Lamnae

HEAT CLEARING
Plum Nelumbinis
Fr Gardenia
Fel Ursi
Rz Anemarrhenae
Hb Lophatheri
Gypsum Fibrosum
Calcitum
Citru Vulgaris
Fo Nelumbinis

DAMP HEAT CLEARING
Rx Gentianae
Rx Scutellariae
Rx Sophorae Flaven.
Cx Phellodendri
Rz Coptidis
Sm Dolichoris
Sm Sojae Germinatum

BLOOD COOLING
Rx Rehmanniae
Rx Scrophularia
Cx Moutan Rx

Rx Macrotomiae
 seu Lithospermi
Rz Imperatae
Cornu Rhinoceri

FALSE HEAT CLEARING
Hb Artemisiae Chin.
Cx Lycii Rx
Rx Cynanchi Atrati
Rx Stellariae

HEAT CLEARING ANTITOXIN
Rx Pulsatillae
Cx dictamni
Fr Forsythiae
Rx Isatidis
Fm Isatidis
Fl Lonicerae
Rz Smilacis
Rx Echinopiae
Rx Sophorae Subst.
Hb Taraxaci
Rx Ampelosis
Rz Belamcandae

HEAT CLEARING EYE BRIGHTENING
Sm Cassiae
Spica Prunellae
Rz Phragmitis
Excrementum
 Vespertili

ANTIMALARIAL
Hb Artemisia Chin.

COLD PHLEGM RESOLVING
Rx Platycodi
Sm Sinapis alba
Spina Gleditsiae
Rz Pinelliae
Rz Arisaematis
Rx Aconiti coreani
Rz Cynanchi Stauto.
Fl Inulae

HEAT PHLEGM RESOLVING
Pumice
Rx Peucedani
Bulbus Fritillaria
 Cirrhosae
Bulbus Fritillaria
 Thunbergii
Bambusa in Taenia
Rx Adenophorae
Rx Trichosanthis

Fr Trichosanthis
Sm Trichosanthis
Succus Bambusae
Hb laminariae
Sargassum
Lpis Chloriti

ANTI-TUSSIVE ANTI-ASTHMATIC
Fl Farfarae
Fr Perilla
Rx Stemonae
Rx Asteris
Cx Mori Rx
Fr Aristolochia
Sm Armeniacae
Fm Eriobotryae

AROMATIC DAMP RESOLVING
Fr seu Sm Amomi
Fr Amomi Cardamomi
Fr Amomi Tsaoko
Sm alpiniae Katsum.
Rz Atractylodis La.
Cx Magnoliae Off.
Hb Agastaches

DIGESTIVE
Massa Fermantata
Fr Oryzae
Fr Hordei
Endo Galli
Sm Raphani
Fr Cratagi

CARMINATIVE
Pericarp. Citri
 Reticulata
Peri. Cit. Reti-
 culata viride
Bulbus Allium
Rx Saussureae
Fr Citri
 Sarcodactylis
Lignum Aquilaria
Rx Linderae
Lignum Santali
Sm Litchi
Peri. Arecae
Fr Ponciri
Fr Aurantii
Rz Cyperi
Calyx Kaki
Fr Meliae Toosen.

PURGATIVE
Rz Rhei
Hb Aloes
Fm Sennae

Mirabilitum
Sm Ricini

LUBRICANT
Sm Cannabis
Sm Pruni

CATHARTIC DIURETIC
Sm Crotonis
Sm Euphorbia Lathy.
Hb Euphorbia Pekin.
Rx Euphorbia Kansui
Sm Pharbitidis
Rx Phytolaccae

ANTIHELMINTHIC
Sm Arecae
Fr Quisqualis
Sm Hydnocarpi
Lythargyrum
Melanteritum
Sm Torreyae
Calomelas
Nidus Vespae

AROMATIC STIMULANT
Rz Acori Gramini
Moschus
Styrax Liquidis
Benzoinum
borneolum
Calculus Bovis

INTERIOR WARMING
Fr Piperis Longae
Fr Piperis
Rz alpiniae Off.
Rz Zingiberis (dry)
Cx Cinnamomi
Rx Aconiti Carmich.
Fr Evodiae
Fr Foeniculi
Fl Caryophylli
Fr Zanthoxyli

LIVER WIND CALMING
Lumbricus
Cornu Antelopis
Concha Haliotidis
Scolopendra
Rz Gastrodia
Fr Tribuli
Scorpio
Bombyx Batryticatus
Rm Uncarriae

LIVER YANG
SEDATIVE
Magnetitum
Margaritifera
Os Draconis
Hematitum
Concha Ostrea

SPIRIT
TRANQUILIZING
Sm Biota
Fl Albizziae
Caulis Polygoni
 Multiflori
Sm Zizyphi Spinosa
Cinnabaris
Rx Polygalae

ANTIHYDROPIC
DIURETIC
Poria cocos
Grifolia
Rz Alismatis
Sm coicis
Sm Benincasae
Rx Stephaniae
Stylus Zeae

URINARY SOOTHE
DIURETIC
Talcum
Medulla Junci
Sm Malvae
Sm Plantaginis
Fr Kochiae
hb Polygoni Avicu.
Hb Dianthi
Hb Pyrrosiae
Caulis Akebiae
Rx Dioscorea Bishie

JAUNDICE
RELIEVING
DIURETIC
Hb Artemisia Capil.

ANTIRHEUMATIC
MUSCLE LAYER
Rx Clematis
Rx Gentianae Macro.
Fr Xanthii
Rx Angelica Tuhuo
Cx Erythrinae

ANTIRHEUMATIC
CHANNEL LAYER
Rx Aconiti Agre
Hb Siegesbeckia
Fr Chaenomelis
Rm Mori

ANTIRHEUMATIC
BONES & TENDONS
Rx Acanthopanacis
Rx Dipsaci
Os Tigris
Agkistrodon

ASTRINGENT
HEMOSTATIC
Rz Bletillae
Hb Agrimoniae
Crinis Carbonisat.

BLOOD COOLING
HEMOSTATIC
Rx Sanguisorbae
Fl Sophorae
Baucumen Biotae
Hb Cirsii Japonica

UNOBSTRUCTING
HEMOSTATIC
Rx Pseudoginseng
Pollen Typhae

CHANNEL WARMING
HEMOSTATIC
Fm Artemisia Argyi

BLOOD INVIGORATING
Rz Curcuma Longae
Rx Curcuma
Rz Zedoariae
Rz Corydalis
Cummi Olibanum
Rz Ligustici Walli.
Fl Carthami
Hb Lycopi
Fr Liquidamberis
Rz Scirbii
 (Sparganii)
Sm Persicae
Commiphora Myrrha
Hb Leonuri
Hb Patriniae
Rx Salviae
Rx Rubiae
Rx Achyranthis
Pyritum
Lignum Sappan
Rx Paeoniae Rubra
Faeces
Trogopterorum
Fr Rosae Chinensis
Succinum
Resina Draconis
Squama Manitis
Sm Vaccariae
Mylabris
Concha Arecae

QI TONIC
Rz Atractylodes
 Alba
Fr Zizyphi Sativae
Rx Glycyrrhizae
Rx Polygonati
Rx Dioscorreae
Rx Codonopsis
Rx Astragali
Saccharum Granorum
Rx Ginseng

YANG TONIC
Rz Drynariae
Rx Dipsaci
Sm Trigonellae
Cornu Cervi
 Pantotrichum
Hippocampus
Sm Cuscutae
Rx Morindae
Cx Eucommiae
Rx Cibotii
Hb Epimedii
Fr Alpiniae Oxylph.
Fr Psoralaeae
Sm allii Tuberosi
Cordyceps
Gecko
Hb cistanches
Sm Juglandis
Hb Cynomori
Rz Cuculiginis
Placenta Hominis

BLOOD TONIC
Rx Angelica
Arillus Longana
Rx Rehmannia Prep.
Fr Mori
Rx Polygoni Multif.
Gelatinum Asini
Fr Lycii
Rx Paeoniae alba

YIN TONICS
Rx Glehniae
Rz Polygonati Off.
Bulbus Lilii
Hb Dendrobi
Rx Ophiopogonis
Rx Panacis
Rx Asparagi
Fr Ligustri
Rm Loranthi
Carapax Amydae
Plastrum
 Testudinis
Sm Sesame
Mel

UPPER JIAO
ASTRINGENT
Fr Tritici
Rx Ephedrae

MIDDLE JIAO
ASTRINGENT
Galla Chinensis
Sm Myristicae
Halloysitum Rubra
Peri. Granati
Fr Chebulae
Cx Ailanthi
Fr Mume
Fr Papaveris

LOWER JIAO
ASTRINGENT
Fr Schisandrae
Fr Corni
Fr Rubi
Os Sepiae
Sm Ginkgo
Fr Rosae Laevigata
Sm Nelumbinis
Sm Eurayles

TOPICAL
Alumen
Fr Cnidii
Sulphur
Caulis Cinnamomi
Secretio Bufonis
Sm Strychni
Catechu Gambier
Borax

EMETIC
Rx Veratri
Calyx Melonis

INDEX A: HERBS BY PHARMACEUTICAL NAME

INDEX B: HERBS BY CHINESE PIN YIN NAME

MATERIALS ON NATURAL HEALTH, ARTS AND SCIENCES

BOOKS

Yellow Emperor's Classic of Medicine By Maoshing Ni, Ph.D.
The *Neijing* is one of the most important classics of Taoism, as well as the highest authority on traditional Chinese medicine. Written in the form of a discourse between Yellow Emperor and his ministers, this book contains a wealth of knowledge on holistic medicine and how human life can attune itself to receive natural support. BYELLO Paperback, 316 p. $16.00

The Tao of Nutrition by Maoshing Ni, Ph.D., with Cathy McNease, B.S., M.H. - This book offers both a healing and a disease prevention system through eating habits. This volume contains 3 major sections: theories of Chinese nutrition and philosophy; descriptions of 100 common foods with energetic properties and therapeutic actions; and nutritional remedies for common ailments. 214 pages, Paperback, Stock No. BNUTR, $14.50

Power of Natural Healing
Hua-Ching Ni discusses the natural capability of self-healing, information and practices which can assist any treatment method and presents methods of cultivation which promote a healthy life, longevity and spiritual achievement. 230 pages, Paperback, Stock No. BHEAL, $14.95

101 Vegetarian Delights by Lily Chuang and Cathy McNease
A vegetarian diet is a gentle way of life with both physical and spiritual benefits. The Oriental tradition provides helpful methods to assure that a vegetarian diet is well-balanced and nourishing. This book provides a variety of clear and precise recipes ranging from everyday nutrition to exotic and delicious feasts. 176 pages, Paperback, Stock No. B101V, $12.95

Chinese Vegetarian Delights by Lily Chuang
An extraordinary collection of recipes based on principles of traditional Chinese nutrition. For those who require restricted diets or who choose an optimal diet, this cookbook is a rare treasure. Meat, sugar, diary products and fried foods are excluded. 104 pages, Paperback, Stock No. BCHIV, $7.50

Strength From Movement: Cultivating Chi by Hua-Ching Ni, Daoshing Ni and Maoshing Ni. *Chi,* the vital power of life, can be developed and cultivated within yourself to help support your health and your happy life. This book gives the deep reality of different useful forms of *chi* exercise and why certain types are more beneficial for certain types of people. Included are samples of several popular exercises. 256 pages, Paperback with 42 photographs, Stock No. BSTRE, $16.95.

Attune Your Body with Dao-In by Hua-Ching Ni
The ancients discovered that Dao-In exercises solved problems of stagnant energy, increased their health and lengthened their years. The exercises are also used as practical support for cultivation and higher achievements of spiritual immortality. 144 pages, Paperback with photographs, Stock No. BDAOI, $14.95 Also on VHS, Stock No. VDAOI, $39.95

Crane Style Chi Gong Book - By Daoshing Ni, Ph.D.
Chi Gong is a set of meditative exercises developed thousands of years ago in China and now practiced for healing purposes. It combines breathing techniques, body movements and mental imagery to guide the smooth flow of energy throughout the body. It may be used with or without the videotape. 55 pages. Stock No. BCRAN. Spiral-bound, $10.95

VIDEO TAPES (VHS)

Self-Healing Chi Gong - By Dr. Maoshing Ni
Many *chi gong* exercises are designed for general health improvement and maintenance, but Self-Healing *Chi Gong* is specifically therapeutic. Self-Healing *Chi Gong* can be applied by a person experiencing disequilibrium in order to restore balance. It consists of specific exercises for each organ system of the body. They are basic and simple, and the effects are immediate. Stock No. VSHCH, $39.95

Attune Your Body with Dao-In - by Master Hua-Ching Ni. Dao-In is a series of movements traditionally used for conducting physical energy. The ancients discovered that Dao-In exercise solves problems of stagnant energy, increases health and lengthens one's years, providing support for cultivation and higher achievements of spiritual immortality. Stock No. VDAOI, VHS $39.95

Eight Treasures - By Maoshing Ni, Ph.D.
These exercises help open blocks in your energy flow and strengthen your vitality. It is a complete exercise combining physical stretching, toning and energy-conducting movements coordinated with breathing. Patterned from nature, its 32 movements are an excellent foundation for T'ai Chi Ch'uan or martial arts. 1 hour, 45 minutes. Stock No. VEIGH. $39.95

T'ai Chi Ch'uan: An Appreciation - by Hua-Ching Ni.
Master Ni presents three styles of T'ai Chi handed down to him through generations of highly developed masters. "Gentle Path," "Sky Journey" and "Infinite Expansion" are presented uninterrupted in this unique videotape, set to music for observation and appreciation. Stock No. VAPPR. VHS 30 minutes $24.95

Crane Style Chi Gong - by Dr. Daoshing Ni, Ph.D.
Chi Gong is a set of meditative exercises practiced for healing chronic diseases, strengthening the body and spiritual enlightenment. Correct and persistent practice will increase one's energy, relieve tension, improve concentration, release emotional stress and restore general well-being. 2 hours, Stock No. VCRAN. $39.95

T'ai Chi Ch'uan I & II - By Maoshing Ni, Ph.D.
This exercise integrates the flow of physical movement with that of internal energy in the Taoist style of "Harmony," similar to the long form of Yang-style T'ai Chi Ch'uan. T'ai Chi has been practiced for thousands of years to help both physical longevity and spiritual cultivation. 1 hour each. Each videotape $39.95. Order both for $69.95. Stock Nos: Part I, VTAI1; Part II, VTAI2; Set of two, VTAI3.

Movement Arts for Emotional Health
Interview of Hua-Ching Ni in the show "Asian-American Focus" hosted by Lili Chu. Dialogue on emotional health and energy exercises that are fundamental to health and well-being. Stock No. VMOVE 30 minutes $15.95

Natural Living and the Universal Way
Interview of Hua-Ching Ni in the show "Asian American Focus" hosted by Lili Chu. Dialogue on common issues of everyday life and practical wisdom. VINTE 30 minutes $15.95

AUDIO CASSETTES

Stress Release with Chi Gong - By Maoshing Ni, Ph.D.
This audio cassette guides you through simple, ancient breathing exercises that enable you to release day-to-day stress and tension that are such a common cause of illness today. 30 minutes. Stock No. ACHIS. $9.95

Pain Management with Chi Gong - By Maoshing Ni, Ph.D.
Using easy visualization and deep-breathing techniques developed over thousands of years, this audio cassette offers methods for overcoming pain by invigorating your energy flow and unblocking obstructions that cause pain. 30 minutes, Stock No. ACHIP. $9.95

Invocations for Health, Longevity and Healing a Broken Heart - By Maoshing Ni, Ph.D. This audio cassette guides the listener through a series of ancient invocations to channel and conduct one's own healing energy and vital force. "Thinking is louder than thunder. The mystical power which creates all miracles is your sincere practice of this principle." 30 minutes, Stock No. AINVO, $9.95

***Tao Teh Ching* Cassette Tapes**
This classic work of Lao Tzu has been recorded in this two-cassette set that is a companion to the book translated by Hua-Ching Ni. Professionally recorded and read by Robert Rudelson. 120 minutes. Stock No. ATAOT. $12.95

POCKET BOOKLETS

Guide to Your Total Well-Being
Simple useful practices for self-development, aid for your spiritual growth and guidance for all aspects of life. Exercise, food, sex, emotional balancing, meditation. 48 pages, paperback, BWELL, $4.00

Less Stress, More Happiness
Helpful information for identifying and relieving stress in your life, including useful techniques such as invocation, breathing and relaxation, meditation, exercise, nutrition and lifestyle balancing. 48 pages, paperback BLESS $3.00

Progress Along the Way: Life, Service and Realization
The guiding power of human life is the association between the developed mind and the achieved soul which contains love, rationality, conscience, and everlasting value. 64 pages, paperback, BPROG $4.00

Integral Nutrition
Nutrition is an integral part of a healthy, balanced life. Includes information on how to asses your basic body type food preparation, energetic properties of food, nutrition and digestion. 32 pages, paperback, BNUTR $3.00

BOOKS IN ENGLISH BY MASTER NI

PERSONAL USEFUL AND PRACTICAL DEVELOPMENT

Self-Reliance and Constructive Change
Natural spiritual reality is independent of concept. Thus, dependency upon religious convention, cultural notions and political ideals must be given up to reach full spiritual potential. The DeClaration of Spiritual Independence affirms spiritual self-authority and true wisdom as the highest attainments of life. 64 pages, paperback, BSELF $7.00

Harmony - The Art of Life
Harmony occurs when two different things find the point at which they can link together. Master Ni shares valuable spiritual understanding and insight about the ability to bring harmony within one's own self, one's relationships and the world. 208 pages, Paperback, Stock No. BHARM, $14.95

Esoteric Tao Teh Ching
Tao Teh Ching expresses the highest efficiency of life and can be applied in many levels of worldly life and spiritual life. This previously unreleased edition discusses instruction for spiritual practices in every day life, which includes important in-depth techniques for spiritual benefit. 192 pages, Paperback, Stock No. BESOT, $12.95

Moonlight in the Dark Night
To attain inner clarity and freedom of the soul, you have to control your emotions. This book contains wisdom on balancing the emotions, including balancing love relationships, so that spiritual achievement becomes possible. 168 pages, Paperback, Stock No. BMOON, $12.95

Internal Growth through Tao
Hua-Ching Ni teaches the more subtle, much deeper sphere of the reality of life that is above the shallow sphere of external achievement. He also clears the confusion caused by some spiritual teachings and guides you in the direction of developing spiritually by growing internally. 208 pages, Paperback, Stock No. BINTE, $13.95

The Mystical Universal Mother
An understanding of both masculine and feminine energies are crucial to understanding oneself, in particular for people moving to higher spiritual evolution. Master Hua-Ching Ni focuses upon the feminine through the examples of some ancient and modern women. 240 pages, Paperback, Stock No. BMYST, $14.95

SPIRITUAL CLASSICS

The Book of Changes and the Unchanging Truth
The legendary classic *I Ching* is recognized as the first written book of wisdom. Leaders and sages throughout history have consulted it as a trusted advisor which reveals the appropriate action in any circumstance. Includes over 200 pages of background material on natural energy cycles, instruction and commentaries. 669 pages, Stock No. BBOOK, Hardcover, $35.00

The Complete Works of Lao Tzu
The *Tao Teh Ching* is one of the most widely translated and cherished works of literature. Its timeless wisdom provides a bridge to the subtle spiritual truth and aids harmonious and peaceful living. Also included is the *Hua Hu Ching*, a later work of Lao Tzu which was lost to the general public for a thousand years. 212 pages, Paperback, Stock No. BCOMP, $12.95

Workbook for Spiritual Development
This material summarizes thousands of years of traditional teachings and little-known practices for spiritual development. There are sections on ancient invocations, natural celibacy and postures for energy channeling. Master Ni explains basic attitudes and knowledge that supports spiritual practice. 240 pages, Paperback, Stock No. BWORK, $14.95

The Taoist Inner View of the Universe
Master Hua-Ching Ni has given all the opportunity to know the vast achievement of the ancient unspoiled mind and its transpiercing vision. This book offers a glimpse of the inner world and immortal realm known to achieved ones and makes it understandable for students aspiring to a more complete life. 218 pages, Paperback, Stock No. BTAOI, $14.95

Tao, the Subtle Universal Law
Most people are unaware that their thoughts and behavior evoke responses from the invisible net of universal energy. To lead a good stable life is to be aware of the universal subtle law in every moment of our lives. This book presents practical methods that have been successfully used for centuries to accomplish this. 208 pages, Paperback, Stock No. BTAOS, $9.95

Ageless Counsel for Modern Life
These sixty-four writings, originally illustrative commentaries on the *I Ching*, are meaningful and useful spiritual guidance on various topics to enrich your life. Hua Ching Ni's delightful poetry and some teachings of esoteric Taoism can be found here as well. 256 pages, Paperback, Stock No. BAGEL, $15.95.

NEW PUBLICATIONS

Gate to Infinity -People who have learned spiritual through years without real progress will be thoroughly guided by the important discourse in this book. Master ni also gives his Dynamic Meditation. Editors recommend that all serious spiritual students who wish to increase their spiritual potency read this one. 208 pages, paperback, BGATE $13.95

Concourse of all Spiritual Paths - All religions, in spite of their surface differences, in their essence return to the great oneness. Hua-Ching Ni looks at what traditional religions offer us today and suggest how to go beyond differences to discover the depth of universal truth. 194 pages, paperback, BCONC, $15.95

The Way, the Truth and the Light
This is the story of the first sage who introduced the way to the world. The life of this young sage links the spiritual achievement of East and West and demonstrates the great spiritual virtue of his love to all people. 232 pages, Paperback, Stock No. BLIGH, $14.95

FUNDAMENTAL READINGS

The Time Is Now for a Better Life and a Better World
The purpose of achievement is on one hand to serve individual self-preservation and also to exercise one's attainment from spiritual cultivation to help all others. It is expected to save the difficulties of the time, to prepare ourselves to create a bright future for the human race and to overcome our modern-day spiritual dilemma by conjoint effort. 136 pages, Paperback, Stock No. BTIME, $10.95

Golden Message - A Guide to Spiritual Life with Self-Study Program for Learning the Integral Way
This volume begins with a traditional treatise by Daoshing and Maoshing Ni about the broad nature of spiritual learning and its application for human life. It is followed by a message from Hua-Ching Ni. An outline of the Spiritual Self-Study Program and Correspondence Course of the College of Tao is included. 160 pages, Paperback, Stock No. BGOLD, $11.95

The Key to Good Fortune: Refining Your Spirit
Straighten Your Way *(Tai Shan Kan Yin Pien)* and The Silent Way of Blessing *(Yin Chia Wen)* are the main guidance for a mature, healthy life. Spiritual improvement can be an integral part of realizing a Heavenly life on earth. 144 pages, Paperback, Stock No. BKEYT, $12.95

Stepping Stones for Spiritual Success
In this volume, Master Ni has taken the best of the traditional teachings and put them into contemporary language to make them more relevant to our time, culture and lives. 160 pages, Paperback, Stock No. BSTEP, $12.95.

The Gentle Path of Spiritual Progress
This book offers a glimpse into the dialogues between a master and his students. In a relaxed, open manner, Master Ni, Hua-Ching explains to his students the fundamental practices that are the keys to experiencing enlightenment in everyday life. 290 pages, Paperback, Stock No. BGENT, $12.95.

Spiritual Messages from a Buffalo Rider, A Man of Tao
Our buffalo nature rides on us, whereas an achieved person rides the buffalo. Hua-Ching Ni gives much helpful knowledge to those who are interested in improving their lives and deepening their cultivation so they too can develop beyond their mundane beings. 242 pages, Paperback, Stock No. BSPIR, $12.95.

8,000 Years of Wisdom, Volume I and II
This two-volume set contains a wealth of practical, down-to-earth advice given by Master Hua-Ching Ni over a five-year period. Drawing on his training in Traditional Chinese Medicine, Herbology and Acupuncture, Hua-Ching Ni gives candid answers to questions on many topics. Volume I includes dietary guidance; 236 pages; Stock No. BWIS1 Volume II includes sex and pregnancy guidance; 241 pages; Stock No. BWIS2. Paperback. Volume I $18.50; Volume II, $12.50

THE WISDOM OF THREE MASTERS

The Way of Integral Life
This book includes practical and applicable suggestions for daily life, philosophical thought, esoteric insight and guidelines for those aspiring to serve the world. The ancient sages' achievement can assist the growth of your own wisdom and balanced, reasonable life. 320 pages, Paperback, Stock No. BWAYS, $14.00. Hardcover, Stock No. BWAYH, $20.00.

Enlightenment: Mother of Spiritual Independence
The inspiring story and teachings of Master Hui Neng, the father of Zen Buddhism and Sixth Patriarch of the Buddhist tradition, highlight this volume. Hui Neng was a person of ordinary birth, intellectually unsophisticated, who achieved himself to become a spiritual leader. 264 pages, Paperback, Stock No. BENLS, $12.50 Hardcover, Stock No. BENLH, $22.00.

Attaining Unlimited Life
Chuang Tzu was perhaps the greatest philosopher and master of Tao. He touches the organic nature of human life more deeply and directly than do other great teachers. This volume also includes questions by students and answers by Master Hua-Ching Ni. 467 pages, Paperback, Stock No. BATTS $18.00; Hardcover, Stock No. BATTH, $25.00.

METAPHYSICAL AND ESOTERIC TEACHING

Internal Alchemy: The Natural Way to Immortality
Ancient spiritually achieved ones used alchemical terminology metaphorically for human internal energy transformation. Internal alchemy intends for an individual to transform one's emotion and lower energy to be higher energy and to find the unity of life in order to reach the divine immortality. 288 pages, Paperback, Stock No. BALCH, $15.95

Mysticism: Empowering the Spirit Within
For more than 8,000 years, mystical knowledge has been passed down by sages. Master Hua-Ching Ni introduces spiritual knowledge of the developed ones which does not use the senses or machines like scientific knowledge, yet can know both the entirety of the universe and the spirits. 200 pages, Paperback, Stock No. BMYST2, $13.95

Guide to Inner Light
Drawing inspiration from the experience of the ancient achieved ones, modern people looking for the true source and meaning of life can find great teachings to direct and benefit them. The invaluable ancient development can teach us to reach the attainable spiritual truth and point the way to the Inner Light. 192 pages, Paperback, Stock No. BGUID, $12.95

Eternal Light
Master Hua-Ching Ni presents the life and teachings of his father, Grandmaster Ni, Yo San, who was a spiritually achieved person, healer and teacher, and a source of inspiration to Master Ni. Some deeper teachings and insights on living a spiritual life and higher achievement are given. 208 pages, Paperback, Stock No. BETER, $14.95

Quest of Soul
Hua-Ching Ni addresses many concepts about the soul such as saving the soul, improving the soul's quality, the free soul, what happens at death and the universal soul. He guides and inspires the reader into deeper self-knowledge and to move forward to increase personal happiness and spiritual depth. 152 pages, Paperback, Stock No. BQUES, $11.95

Life and Teaching of Two Immortals, Volume 2: Chen Tuan
The second emperor of the Sung Dynasty entitled Master Chen Tuan "Master of Supernatural Truth." Master Ni describes his life and cultivation and gives in-depth commentaries which provide teaching and insight into the achievement of this highly respected Master. 192 pages, Paperback, Stock No. BLIF2, $12.95

Life and Teaching of Two Immortals, Volume 1: Kou Hong
Master Kou Hong was an achieved Master, a healer in Traditional Chinese Medicine and a specialist in the art of refining medicines who was born in 363 A.D. He laid the foundation of later cultural development in China. 176 pages, Paperback, Stock No. BLIF1, $12.95.

The Story of Two Kingdoms
This volume is the metaphoric tale of the conflict between the Kingdoms of Light and Darkness. Through this unique story, Master Ni transmits esoteric teachings of Taoism which have been carefully guarded secrets for over 5,000 years. This book is for those who are serious in achieving high spiritual goals. 122 pages, Stock No. BSTOR, Hardcover, $14.50

Seven✪Star Mail Order Form

Name: _____

Address: _____

City: _____ State: _____ Zip: _____

Phone (daytime): _____ (Evening): _____

Qty.	Stock #	Title	Price ea.	Subtotal

Sales tax (CA residents only): _____

Shipping: _____

Total: _____

Payment: Check, money order or credit card

Card number: _____

Exp. date

Signature: _____

Shipping: via UPS in the continental United States. $5.50 for first item and 50¢ for each additional item. The *I Ching* counts as 3 items. Please call for international shipping rates to all other locations.

Telephone orders, questions or catalog requests: 800/578-9526
Website: www.taostar.com   E-mail: taostar@taostar.com

Mail form with payment (US funds only) to:
13315 Washington Blvd. Suite 200 • Los Angeles, California 90066

Herbs Used by Ancient Masters

The pursuit of everlasting youth or immortality throughout human history is an innate human desire. Long ago, Chinese esoteric Taoists went to the high mountains to contemplate nature, strengthen their bodies, empower their minds and develop their spirit. From their studies and cultivation, they China alchemy and chemistry, herbology and acupuncture, the I Ching, astrology, martial arts and T'ai Chi Ch'uan, Chi Gong and many other useful kinds of knowledge.

Most important, they handed down in secrecy methods for attaining longevity and spiritual immortality. There were different levels of approach; one was to use a collection of food herb formulas that were only available to highly achieved Taoist masters. They used these food herbs to increase energy and heighten vitality. This treasured collection of herbal formulas remained within the Ni family for centuries.

Now, through Traditions of Tao, the Ni family makes these foods available for you to use to assist the foundation of your own positive development. It is only with a strong foundation that expected results are produced from diligent cultivation. For further information about Traditions of Tao herbal products, please call or mail this form to:

Traditions of Tao
13315 Washington Boulevard Suite 200
Los Angeles, CA 90066
(800) 772-0222

Please send me a Traditions of Tao brochure!

Name_____

Address _____

City _____ State _____ Zip_____

Phone (day) _____ (evening) _____

- -

Yo San University of Traditional Chinese Medicine
"Not just a medical career, but a life-time commitment to raising one's spiritual standard."

Thank you for your support and interest in our publications and services. It is by your patronage that we continue to offer you the practical knowledge and wisdom from this venerable Taoist tradition.

Because of your sustained interest in Taoism, in January 1989 we formed Yo San University of Traditional Chinese Medicine, a non-profit educational institution under the direction of founder Master Ni, Hua-Ching. Yo San University is the continuation of 38 generations of Ni family practitioners who handed down knowledge and wisdom from father to son. Its purpose is to train and graduate practitioners of the highest caliber in Traditional Chinese Medicine, which includes acupuncture, herbology and spiritual development.

We view Traditional Chinese Medicine as the application of spiritual development. Its foundation is the spiritual capability to know life, to diagnose a person's problem and how to cure it. We teach students how to care for themselves and others, emphasizing the integration of traditional knowledge and modern science. Yo San University offers a complete Master's degree program approved by the California State Department of Education that provides an excellent education in Traditional Chinese Medicine and meets all requirements for state licenser.

We invite you to inquire into our university for a creative and rewarding career as a holistic physician. Classes are also open to persons interested only in self-enrichment. For more information, please fill out the form below and send it to:

Yo San University
of Traditional Chinese Medicine
13315 Washington Boulevard Suite 200
Los Angeles, CA 90066

❑ Please send me information on the Masters degree program in Traditional Chinese Medicine.
❑ Please send me information on health workshops and seminars.
❑ Please send me information on continuing education for acupuncturists and health professionals.

Name_____

Address _____

City _____ State _____ Zip_____

Phone (day) _____ (evening) _____

Spiritual Study and Teaching Through the College of Tao

The College of Tao and SevenStar Communications were formally established in California in the 1970's, yet this tradition is a very old spiritual culture containing centuries of human spiritual growth. Its central goal is to offer healthy spiritual education to all people. This time-tested school values the spiritual development of each individual self and passes down its guidance and experience.

The College of Tao is a school which has no walls. The greater human society is its classroom. Your own teaching and service is the class you attend; thus students grow from their lives and from studying the guidance of the Integral Way. The goal of the school is to help individuals develop themselves and become Mentors of the Integral Way. A Mentor is any individual who is spiritually self-responsible and who sets up the model of a healthy and complete life for oneself and others.

Any interested individual is welcome to join and learn to grow for oneself. The Correspondence Course/Self-Study Program can be useful to you. The Program, which is based on Master Ni's books and videotapes, gives people who wish to study on their own or are too far from a center or volunteer teachers, an opportunity to study the learning of the Way at their own speed. The outline of how to participate in the Correspondence Course/Self-Study Program can be found at the end of the book, *The Golden Message*.

It is recommended that all Mentors of the Integral Way use the self-study program in *The Golden Message* to educate themselves. They can teach special skills which are certified by the College of Tao. Those who engage in teaching with Master Ni's materials must follow the Mentor Service Regulations of the College of Tao. To receive recognition from the College of Tao for teaching activity, a Mentor must register with the College.

If you are interested in the Universal Society of the Integral Way Correspondence Course/Self-Study Program, please write: College of Tao • PO Box 1222 • El Prado, NM 87529

Mail to: USIW • 13315 Washington Blvd., Suite 200 • Los Angeles, CA 90066

_____ I wish to be put on the mailing list of the USIW to be notified of educational activities.
_____ I wish to receive a list of registered Mentors teaching in my area or country.
_____ I am interested in joining/forming a study group in my area.
_____ I am interested in becoming a Mentor of the USIW.

Name _____

Address _____

City _____ State _____ Zip _____